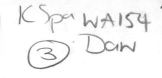
EMQs for the nMRCGP® Applied Knowledge Test

with answers discussed

Second Edition

Hayley Dawson MBBS DRCOG DFFP MRCGP

and

Anna Trigell BA MBBS MRCGP DRCOG DCH DFFP Dip Clin Derm

Radcliffe Publishing

Oxford • New York

Radcliffe Publishing Ltd
18 Marcham Road
Abingdon
Oxon OX14 1AA
United Kingdom

www.radcliffe-oxford.com
Electronic catalogue and worldwide online ordering facility.

British Library Cataloguing in Publication Data

A catalogue record for this book is available from the British Library.

ISBN-13: 978 184619 245 6

Typeset by Duck Creations, Ducklington, Oxon
Printed and bound by TJI Digital, Padstow, Cornwall

Contents

iv   Contents

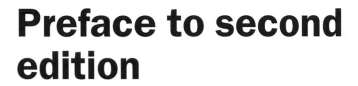

Preface to second edition

The MRCGP® exam and Summative Assessment have now merged to become the compulsory nMRCGP® and with this has come a change in the format of the written exam. Rather than Paper 1 and Paper 2 there is now a single Applied Knowledge Test consisting of one three hour exam. There has also been a move to computer based tests, so hopefully, no more confusion with question numbering.

The questions themselves remain similar in format, but we have updated this edition to include revised guidelines and added in some questions on relatively new topics such as practice-based commissioning.

Hayley Dawson
Anna Trigell
April 2008

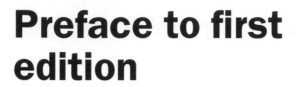

Preface to first edition

We have written this book as we were somewhat taken by surprise by the recent changes in the Summative Assessment MCQ exam and the MRCGP® MCQ exam.

In the last few years the question format has changed from the standard true or false MCQs that we know and love, to the more involved and less guessable EMQs (extended matching questions). We have lost negative marking (hurray), as this was found to be a confounding variable when used for assessment.

This book is designed to familiarise you with the types of questions to be found in the new exam, and also to cover good exam technique in order to optimise your results with the knowledge you have.

Hayley Dawson
Anna Trigell
January 2005

About the exam

nMRCGP®

The nMRCGP® is a modular exam with three components. The Applied Knowledge Test (AKT) is a computer-based multiple-choice question exam.

- *Duration*: The exam lasts for three hours.
- *Number of questions*: There are 200 questions.
- *Pass marks*: The pass mark varies between 63% and 70% but the pass rate is good. Approximately eight out of ten people pass, so the chances are that you will be in this majority!

Content of the exam

This is based on the General Medical Council's document *Good Medical Practice* (2001), which sets out seven broad headings as follows.

- Good clinical care.
- Maintaining good medical practice.
- Relationships with patients.
- Working with colleagues.
- Teaching and training, assessment and appraisal.
- Probity.
- Health and the performance of other doctors.

The whole syllabus can be found at www.rcgp.org.uk.

We hope that this book will help to ensure you pass the exam first time.

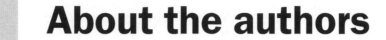

About the authors

Hayley Dawson and **Anna Trigell** qualified from Imperial College School of Medicine in 1999. Hayley joined a vocational training scheme in Barnet, North London, and Anna split her vocational training between St Mary's, Paddington and Addenbrookes, Cambridgeshire. They both sat the MRCGP® Examination in 2003 and both achieved a pass with Merit in the multiple-choice component (Paper 2).

Hayley is working as a GP in North London. Anna is a GP in St Neots, Cambridgeshire and is a GPwSI in dermatology.

Acknowledgements

We would like to thank Vince Mak and Simon Merchant for their patience, and Dr Emma Radcliffe (GP), Drs Penny and Will Zermansky (GPs) and Dr Anders Skarsten (Consultant Psychiatrist) for their assistance with editing. We are also grateful to Gillian Nineham and her team at Radcliffe Publishing.

The illustrations on pp.76–8 are reproduced with permission from Ashton R and Leppard B (2005) *Differential Diagnosis in Dermatology* (3e). Radcliffe Publishing, Oxford.

Good exam technique

1 Revision

This is certainly the hardest exam to revise for as the questions can be about anything. Subjects we suggest should definitely be learned, as they represent easy marks, include the following:

- DVLA exclusion criteria
- benefits (e.g. income support, disability living allowance, etc.)
- mental health Sections
- forms (e.g. Med 3, DS1500, Mat B1)
- child development milestones
- statistics (e.g. sensitivity, specificity, number needed to treat, etc.).

Practise questions as much for timing as for subject matter. This book is designed to help with planning timing, as we have divided the questions into eight papers. You should be aiming to complete each paper within 45 minutes to comply with the exam timing.

It is worth having the above written down on one piece of paper that can be read on the way to the exam. They seem to have a fleeting existence in short-term memory, and however well you learned them two weeks before the exam, it is worth reminding yourself the morning or the night before.

2 Arrive on time

We all know this one. However, there is always a sizeable minority who are rushing from the train/tube/car park with minutes to spare.

Try to allow as much time as you are ever likely to need *and then some more* for travelling to and finding the exam building.

There are 150 Pearson VUE test centres in the UK, so hopefully you won't have to travel too far. The sooner you book your place for the exam the more likely you are to get your exam centre of choice.

Please bear in mind the rules on the Royal College website that stipulate:

'**Late arrivals will not be admitted.**'

3 What to bring

You must bring two identification documents, both with name and signature and at least one with a photo.

You will not be allowed to bring anything into the exam room although you can leave for food, water or the toilet.

4 Read the instructions

This is as important for computer-based testing as it is for written papers, possibly more so as it is a new format.

There is a short tutorial at the start of the exam to explain how to answer the questions. There is also a familiarity tutorial on the Pearson VUE website at www.pearsonvue.co.uk/home/cbt/tutorials

We would strongly recommend spending five minutes running through this as it will be one less thing to worry about on the day, especially if computers are not your forte.

5 Read the question

Check for negatives. Some questions will require you to choose up to three (occasionally more) best answers. Marks are easily lost if the wrong number of answers is given.

6 Strategy

There are many ways in which candidates answer MCQ and EMQ papers. We believe that if you don't know the answer the first time around, you are unlikely to know it half an hour later. By answering the questions you feel confident about and coming back to the rest later, you run the risk of both forgetting that you have to come back to them, thereby automatically losing the marks, and also effectively spending twice as long on some questions (i.e. reading them first and deciding that you don't know the answer and will come back to them, and reading them again to try to answer them). This means you are increasing the risk of running out of time. Our strategy therefore is to answer everything on the first attempt, with the caveat below . . .

7 Timing

The EMQ exam is very wordy, and it is easy to get bogged down by the questions, especially if English is not your first language. It is possible to spend too much time on questions and thus run out of time. Try to calculate how many marks a question is worth, and if you find that you are puzzling for a long time over one question, which is perhaps only worth one mark, then put down your best guess and make a note to come back to it if you have time at the end. This can be especially useful for questions that take some working out, such as ECGs, audiograms and statistics, or very long-winded questions, such as the 'fill in the blanks' type.

In the exam, check timing throughout. Make sure that after an hour of the exam you are at least a third of the way through the questions, and so on. If you are running on schedule, try to build in a two-minute break midway. Stretch, have a small snack, or go to the toilet. It is a long exam and a hard day. It is normal to despair about two-thirds of the way through. Work through this – the end is near. Don't become too concerned if you think you know very little about a question. One strategy is to best-guess it and move on quickly. There is not much point in leaving it to come back to later.

If you don't know it now, it is unlikely that you will know it by the end of the exam – you will just end up wasting more time.

8 Finishing

In the new format exam, you will not be allowed to leave early. Take care if you use this time to recheck your answers as there is some evidence you are more likely to change correct answers.

Good luck . . .

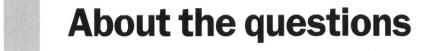

About the questions

The more old-fashioned multiple-choice questions have been gradually phased out in recent years. Although they test factual information, they do not give an indication of the candidate's ability to perform higher-order skills such as data interpretation and problem solving. The current mode of questioning, namely 'extended matching questions', tests material that is relevant to practice and avoids the esoteric (and sometimes interesting) topics that are not essential. The idea is to assess the candidate's information base as well as their ability to utilise that information.

Most of the questions posed in the MRCGP® (and the Step 2 examination and US MLE) provide patient vignettes that focus on tasks relevant to the candidate's day-to-day clinical practice. These will be tasks such as forming likely diagnoses or determining the next step in management. Answering these questions requires interpretation and synthesis of data and application of knowledge to both familiar and unusual clinical situations, which should reflect many of your consultations.

The areas tested should focus on questions appropriate to general practice, so for example they are unlikely to focus on the management of high-risk pregnancies, but are more likely to look at prenatal counselling or uncomplicated antenatal care. They want to ensure that the candidate is capable of a broad spectrum of clinical responsibility while at the same time being able to utilise secondary care services appropriately.

In devising the questions the authors will rarely use real patients, as they are too complicated, and in general 'red herrings' are avoided. Also, although in real life patients may be selective about the truth, the candidate can take the information presented in the questions at face value. An example of this would be the patient with a hacking cough who smokes five cigarettes a week – if that is what the question says, look for the answer appropriate to the information given.

In deciding the clinical content of the question, the authors of the exam are given the following guidelines.

1 Use clinical vignettes to test the candidate's clinical decision-making skills.
2 Focus on either the common or the potentially catastrophic problems essential to competent practice, and avoid esoterica.
3 Avoid specialist scenarios that would be handled in secondary care.

Examples of typical types of question

What would be the next step in management of the following patients?

Questions may contain lists of medications or investigations. Questions will sometimes be testing the candidate's knowledge of and ability to apply up-to-date guidelines.

What is the likely cause of the following presentations?

Questions may present laboratory results/presentations of clinical problems.

Fill in the gaps

There will be the odd question presenting a paragraph such as a NICE guideline or some text on a subject such as would be found in a clinical textbook.

How to use this book

We have grouped the questions into 'papers', each consisting of 50 questions, which can be used to practise exam timing by giving yourself 45 minutes per paper. The answers can be found at the end of each paper.

Alternatively, you can use this book by referring to the topic-based question index on the following pages. This way you can test yourself on specific subjects to tie in with your revision.

Question index by topic

Assessing quality of care

Benefits, certification and allowances

Cardiology

Dermatology

Paper 2: 43–47
Paper 3: 46–50

Ear, nose and throat

Paper 2: 9–12
Paper 3: 34–38
Paper 4: 9–13, 36–41
Paper 6: 1–4
Paper 7: 35–39
Paper 8: 24–27

Endocrinology

Paper 1: 19
Paper 2: 1–8
Paper 3: 25–27
Paper 4: 14–17
Paper 5: 29–33
Paper 6: 45–49

Ethics

Paper 2: 50
Paper 6: 40
Paper 8: 47–50

Gastroenterology

Paper 1: 6–10
Paper 2: 20–24
Paper 3: 15–19

Neurology

Paper 1: 29–31
Paper 2: 49
Paper 4: 48
Paper 5: 45–47
Paper 6: 19–21
Paper 7: 46–49
Paper 8: 36–40

Ophthalmology

Paper 1: 32–36
Paper 7: 26–30

Paediatrics

Paper 1: 49
Paper 2: 13–17
Paper 3: 39–43
Paper 4: 43–47
Paper 5: 14–18
Paper 6: 5–11
Paper 7: 44
Paper 8: 28–31

Palliative care

Paper 8: 41–44

Pharmacotherapeutics

Psychiatry

Reproductive medicine

Respiratory medicine

Statistics and study design

Paper 3: 20–24
Paper 4: 22–25
Paper 5: 6–13

Urology/Renal medicine

Paper 1: 37–43
Paper 2: 42
Paper 3: 10
Paper 5: 5
Paper 6: 22–24
Paper 7: 25
Paper 8: 8–20, 46

Paper 1 Questions

Theme: The audit cycle

Options:

A   Agree criteria
B   Review available evidence
C   Observe current practice
D   Identify change needed
E   Implement change
F   Monitor the effect of change

Using the above options, complete the following audit cycle:

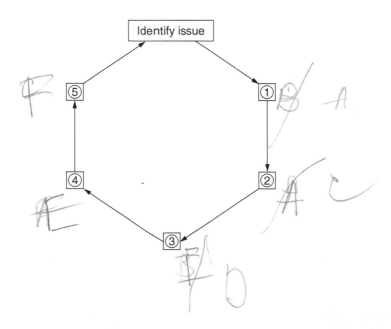

Theme: Dyspepsia

Options:

A ^{13}C urea breath test
B   Full blood count
C   Urgent endoscopy
D   Routine endoscopy
E   Trial of Gaviscon or similar
F   Trial of proton-pump inhibitor
G   Prophylactic proton-pump inhibitor
H   Cox II inhibitor
I   1 week of triple therapy (full dose PPI + 2 antibiotics)
J   2 weeks of triple therapy followed by 2 months of anti-secretory therapy (PPIs)

Choose the most appropriate next step in management for the following patients:

(6)   A 26-year-old man presents with a history of 2 months of retrosternal burning pain, especially at night.   *E*

(7)   A 56-year-old woman has had new-onset retrosternal burning with excessive wind and nausea for the past 6 weeks.

(8)   A 54-year-old man comes to see you after his endoscopy, which demonstrated a *Helicobacter pylori*-positive duodenal ulcer. He was given a prescription at the hospital but misplaced it, and would like you to issue the medications recommended for treatment of his duodenal ulcer.

(9)   A 43-year-old woman who was referred for an endoscopy with anaemia and dyspepsia was found to have a *Helicobacter*-positive gastric ulcer. She has been treated appropriately for this with oral medication. What further management option should occur 6–8 weeks later?

(10) A 62-year-old man has a history of dyspepsia since his mid-thirties. He has no red flag symptoms and tests positive on a stool antigen test for *H. pylori*.

Theme: Psychological treatments

Options:

A   Analytical psychotherapy
B   Behavioural therapy
C   Cognitive therapy
D   Cognitive–behavioural therapy
E   Counselling
F   Crisis therapy
G   Problem solving

For each of the following patient examples, choose the most appropriate type of psychological treatment.

(11) A 34-year-old woman has been on numerous antidepressants over the years, and has had several counselling sessions within the practice. She comes asking for more help, as she is having difficulties maintaining relationships and feels emotionally vulnerable. There is no specific external trigger to the way she is feeling.

(12) A 47-year-old man with chronic, well-controlled schizophrenia has been refusing to answer the phone, has not been eating properly and has been sleeping most of the day since the loss of his mother 2 weeks ago. He has other family nearby who report that he has been extremely withdrawn and tearful. He has lived with his mother all his life.

(13)   A 39-year-old woman has just miscarried for the second time. She is deeply upset and unable to function. She feels that she does not want to burden her husband with the way she is feeling.

(14)   A 7-year-old boy has nocturnal enuresis. Organic pathology has been ruled out. His parents are supportive but desperate to resolve the problem.

Theme: Joint pain

Options:

A   Ankylosing spondylitis
B   Chondrocalcinosis   ✓
C   Enteropathic arthritis
D   Gout
E   Osteoarthrosis
F   Psoriatic arthropathy
G   Reiter's syndrome
H   Rheumatoid arthritis
I   Septic arthritis
J   Systemic lupus erythematosus

What is the likely diagnosis for the following patients with joint trouble?

(15)   A 50-year-old woman presents with an acute inflammatory arthritis of her left knee. She has no preceding joint problems and is otherwise fit and well. An X-ray shows some calcification of the articular surfaces, and aspirated fluid has a negative Gram stain but crystals are seen.

(16)   A 55-year-old man presents with a 1-day history of severe pain and swelling of the right first metatarsophalangeal joint.

(17) An elderly woman presents with a history of several months of increasing pain in her left first carpo-metacarpal joint after a day's gardening. Examination reveals some swelling and tenderness of the joint, as well as swellings over her distal interphalangeal joints, some of which feel cystic in nature and others bony.

(18) A 30-year-old man presents with a 1-week history of bilateral knee swelling. He has had nagging lower back pain for several months, and has been getting abdominal cramps and opening his bowels up to ten times a day for the past 6 weeks.

Theme: Interpretation of blood tests

(19) You are called to see a 78-year-old man who lives alone. He has been unwell for a fortnight, but didn't want to bother anybody. His last visit to the surgery was 15 years ago. He appears quite dehydrated and confused, so you do some tests. The results are shown below.

Blood tests (normal values in brackets):

Glucose	50 mmol/l	(3.5–7)
Sodium	135 mmol/l	(135–145)
Potassium	5.0 mmol/l	(3.5–5)
Urea	19 mmol/l	(2.5–6.7)
Creatinine	145 micromoles/l	(70–140)
Plasma osmolality	349 mosmol/kg	(278–305)
Hb	18 g/l	(13.5–18)
WCC	17×10^9/l	(4–11)
Platelets	268×10^9/l	(150–400)
CRP	70 mg/l	(< 5)

Urine dip

Ketones	++
Leucocytes	+

What is the likely diagnosis?

Options:

A   Dehydration secondary to urinary tract infection
B   Dehydration secondary to self-neglect
C   Renal failure
D   Diabetic ketoacidosis
E   Hyperosmolar non-ketotic state
F   Syndrome of inappropriate ADH secretion
G   Nephrogenic diabetes insipidus

Theme: GMS contract

Options:

A   Global sum
B   Quality and Outcome Framework payments
C   Seniority payments
D   Directed Enhanced Services
E   Premises
F   Enhanced services

Under which of the above categories would you be paid for the following services?

(20) Starting an anticoagulant monitoring clinic that will accept patients from other practices in your primary care trust.

(21) Starting a cardiovascular disease clinic to ensure that you have comprehensive data and monitoring of the practice's affected patients.

(22) You have a somewhat elderly population, so will need extra resources to manage their extra needs.

(23) Your practice already runs contraception clinics, and intends to continue to do so.

Theme: Hypertension guidelines

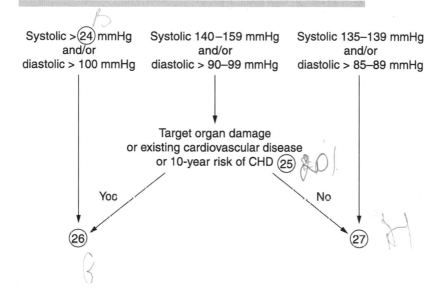

Systolic > (24) mmHg
and/or
diastolic > 100 mmHg

Systolic 140–159 mmHg
and/or
diastolic > 90–99 mmHg

Systolic 135–139 mmHg
and/or
diastolic > 85–89 mmHg

Target organ damage
or existing cardiovascular disease
or 10-year risk of CHD (25)

Yes

No

(26)

(27)

Complete the above flow chart.

A   200
B   160
C   140
D   > 20%
E   > 15%
F   > 30%
G   Treat
H   Reassess annually
I   Reassess 5-yearly
J   No further assessment

Theme: Drugs known to exacerbate psoriasis

(28) Which of the following drugs are known to exacerbate psoriasis? Choose three.

A   Chloroquine
B   Atenolol
C   Lithium
D   Captopril
E   Aspirin
F   Erythromycin
G   Haloperidol

Theme: Tremor

Options:

A   Arterial blood gases
B   Full blood count
C   Liver function tests
D   Lumbar puncture for oligoclonal bands
E   MRI scan
F   Reassure
G   Serum caeruloplasmin
H   Syphilis serology
I   Thyroid function tests
J   Start medication

Which of the above would be the most appropriate next step in management in the following scenarios?

(29) A 35-year-old woman presenting with subfertility also complains of irritability and a fine resting tremor.

(30) A 21-year-old medical student is very concerned that his hands shake when he is trying to perform venous cannulations. He has noticed that alcohol seems to prevent the tremor.

(31) A woman brings her elderly father to see you, concerned that he has 'slowed down'. You note a coarse resting tremor with a frequency of about 4 Hz.

Theme: Red eye

Options:

A   Episcleritis
B   Allergic conjunctivitis
C   Corneal ulcer
D   Trichiasis
E   Acute glaucoma
F   Bacterial conjunctivitis
G   Acute iritis
H   Corneal abrasion
I   Adenoviral conjunctivitis
J   Blepharitis

What is the likely diagnosis for the following patients?

(32) A 24-year-old woman presents with a 1-week history of itching of both eyes. On examination there is lid oedema and chemosis.

(33) An 8-year-old boy is brought to you with a 2-day history of bilateral eye irritation and a watery discharge. On examination you note cobblestoning on the inside lower lids and pre-auricular lymphadenopathy.

(34) A 40-year-old man complains of sudden onset of light hurting his left eye, associated with redness and blurred vision. You note that the pupils are of unequal size.

(35) A 67-year-old woman is seen in the emergency surgery with acute loss of vision, ocular pain, and nausea and vomiting.

(36) A 16-year-old complains of a 1-day history of grittiness and redness in both eyes. Her eyelids were stuck together on waking that morning.

Theme: Urinary incontinence

Options:

A Detrusor instability
B Genuine stress incontinence
C Outflow obstruction
D Urinary tract infection

Match the treatment below with the condition it is used to treat.

(37) Pelvic floor exercises.

(38) Bladder training.

(39) Anticholinergic medication.

(40) Catheterisation.

(41) Antibiotic therapy.

(42) Vaginal cones.

(43) 5-Alpha reductase inhibitors.

Theme: Notifiable diseases

(44) Which three of the following are *not* notifiable diseases?

A   Anthrax
B   Chlamydia
C   Diphtheria
D   Hand, foot and mouth disease
E   HIV
F   Malaria
G   Measles
H   Suspected food poisoning
I   TB
J   Whooping cough

Theme: Tired all the time

Options:

A   Depressive illness
B   Stress
C   Anaemia
D   Acute postviral fatigue
E   Chronic fatigue syndrome
F   Hypothyroidism
G   Hyperthyroidism
H   Heart failure
I   Renal failure
J   Liver failure
K   Malignancy
L   Polymyalgia rheumatica
M   Tuberculosis

Which of the above are the most likely diagnoses for the following
patient vignettes?

(45) A 30-year-old woman presents with tiredness and a 6-month history of increasingly heavy periods since the birth of her second child.

(46) An overweight 73-year-old Asian woman presents with a history of several months of tiredness and breathlessness on exertion. On examination she has pitting oedema of her ankles and fine inspiratory crepitations bibasally.

(47) A 19-year-old student presents with tiredness and difficulty concentrating since a throat infection 3 months previously.

(48) An 84-year-old man presents with a 6-week history of tiredness, weight loss and diarrhoea.

Theme: Neonatal jaundice

(49) Neonatal jaundice can only be said to be physiological if it is present at which time? Choose the single best answer.

A   Day 1
B   Days 2 to 6
C   Days 7 to 14

Theme: Medication (analgesia) in a breastfeeding mother

(50) A 28-year-old woman has recently had a Caesarean section and is currently breastfeeding. She requests some analgesia as the wound site is painful, especially at night.

Which two of the following analgesics would be most suitable?

A   Aspirin
B   Codeine
C   Indomethacin
D   Paracetamol
E   Temazepam

Paper 1 Answers

Theme: The audit cycle

1. A
2. C
3. D
4. E
5. F

Discussion

This question gives you a gentle start. You should be very familiar with the audit process.

Theme: Dyspepsia

6. E
7. C
8. J
9. D
10. I

Discussion

The National Institute for Clinical Excellence (NICE) published guidance on the management of dyspepsia which was updated in June 2005. This guidance can be found at http://guidance.nice.org.

You should be clear in your mind about the management of this common condition.

The current recommendation is 'test (for *H. pylori*) and treat (with proton pump inhibitors)' any patient under 55 years of age with symptoms of dyspepsia, unless there are red flag symptoms such as anaemia or weight loss. Red flag symptoms at any age merit an urgent endoscopy.

Those over 55 years old with recent onset of dyspepsia that has been present for 4–6 weeks should also be referred for urgent endoscopy to exclude malignancy.

Duodenal ulcers are usually adequately treated with one week of triple therapy. Longer treatment courses give slightly higher eradication rates but do not appear cost-effective.

Non-healing gastric ulcers have significant malignant potential, hence the need for further endoscopy 6–8 weeks later to ensure healing has occurred.

The last gentleman does not fulfil the criteria for urgent endoscopy, and eradication therapy would be an appropriate next step, but with a low threshold for further investigation should his symptoms not resolve.

Theme: Psychological treatments

(11) A

(12) F

(13) E

(14) B

Discussion

Analytical psychotherapy is useful for people with longstanding dysthymia that is based on internal triggers.

Crisis therapy should be available for vulnerable people (e.g. those with chronic severe mental illness) when they are confronting life situations that may destabilise them.

Counselling is part of our everyday consultations, and there are other bodies around that may help (e.g. the Miscarriage Association), which can offer counselling tailored to specific situations.

Enuresis alarms are the most effective treatment for nocturnal enuresis. Children are 13 times more likely to achieve 14 consecutive dry nights with alarm treatments than with placebo. The bell and pad technique is an example of an enuresis alarm, and is a form of behavioural therapy that is often used to treat nocturnal enuresis in children. Enuresis alarms are less likely to be successful if the parents are unenthusiastic or if there is a psychological or social instability.

Theme: Joint pain

(15) B
(16) D
(17) E
(18) C

Discussion

A rudimentary knowledge of the various rheumatological conditions is necessary, but the clinical presentations in the exam tend to fit quite obvious patterns of disease.

The differential for the patient described in Question 15 would be any acute swollen joint. Calcium pyrophosphate deposition tends to be slightly less severe than gout, and affects larger joints acutely (e.g. knees/shoulder/wrist).

Osteoarthritis in the hand will often affect the first carpo-metacarpal joint. Heberden's nodes affect the distal interphalangeal joints, and Bouchard's nodes (in rheumatoid arthritis) tend to affect the proximal interphalangeal joints. Osteoarthritis can be managed within general practice, but if rheumatoid arthritis is suspected, early referral to a rheumatologist is indicated, as early treatment with disease-modifying drugs can inhibit progression of the disease.

Theme: Interpretation of blood tests

(19) E

Discussion

Plasma osmolality = [2 × (Na + K) + urea + glucose]

Don't be misled by urinary ketones, as anyone who is unwell/dehydrated/probably not eating is going to be ketotic.

Note that the normal values will nearly always be included, as would happen in real life.

Theme: GMS contract

(20) F
(21) B
(22) A
(23) A

Discussion

The GMS contract was finalised in April 2004. PMS contracts are similar but with locally negotiated terms depending on the population's needs.

The latest government initiatives you may need to know about are 'choice and book', 'electronic prescribing service' and 'practice-based commissioning'.

Theme: Hypertension guidelines

(24) B

(25) D

(26) G

(27) H

Discussion

The British Hypertension Society guidelines were updated in June 2006. The latest guidelines can be found at www.nice.org.uk/CG034.

Theme: Drugs known to exacerbate psoriasis

(28)   A B and C

Discussion

Occasionally psoriasis can be exacerbated or provoked by drugs. The psoriasis may not be seen until the drug has been taken for a number of weeks or even several months. The drugs most commonly associated with such exacerbation are: β-blockers, anti-malarials and lithium.

Theme: Tremor

(29) I

(30) F

(31) J

Discussion

This is a two-stage question. As well as having to work out the diagnosis, you have to decide which is the next most appropriate step in management. Do not try to complicate this. Although in practice one would probably do a number of tests, for the purpose of the exam, once you think you know the condition, find the answer that is most relevant to this.

Try not to fall into the trap of either choosing the gold standard test (e.g. MRI) for everyone, or choosing a common test that would probably be performed on many different presentations (e.g. FBC).

In the above question, the diagnoses are hyperthyroidism (Question 29), benign essential tremor (Question 30) and Parkinson's disease (Question 31). It could be argued that there are other tests one would perform before starting medication for Parkinson's disease, but the history is fairly unequivocal, and none of the other options would be appropriate as the diagnosis is mainly clinical.

Also, while you are revising, try to think of why the other alternatives have been offered. For example, serum caeruloplasmin may seem obscure, but Wilson's disease can present with tremor, as can carbon dioxide retention, alcohol withdrawal, multiple sclerosis, medication, cerebellar ataxia and syphilis.

Theme: Red eye

(32) B

(33) I

(34) G

(35) E
(36) F

Discussion

Fairly technical terminology can be used in this sort of question, and it is worth looking at an ophthalmology textbook to remind yourself of these terms. You may also be given photos of eye conditions to diagnose, including retinal conditions.

Theme: Urinary incontinence

(37) B
(38) A
(39) A
(40) C
(41) D
(42) B
(43) C

Discussion

Revise the differences between detrusor instability and genuine stress incontinence. Urodynamic studies are the only way to differentiate clinically between the two conditions, which coexist in approximately a third of patients.

Theme: Notifiable diseases

(44) B D and E

Discussion

As a rough guide, anything that can be immunised against and all travellers' infections are notifiable. Significant exclusions are the sexually transmitted infections, including HIV (although ophthalmia neonatorum is notifiable). It is also worth noting that questions like this are only worth one mark, so do not agonise over them for too long.

Theme: Tired all the time

 C
46 H
47 D
48 K

Discussion

This is a common presenting complaint in general practice, and it is highly likely to come up in the exam. This is an example of a question where incidental findings have been included but not red herrings. Therefore do not try to read too much into them – they are really not complex.

Theme: Neonatal jaundice

49 B

Discussion

Physiological jaundice is common and occurs because the liver takes over the excretion of bilirubin from the placenta. This usually manifests during days 2–6. Jaundice in the first 24 hours of birth is assumed to be pathological (usually haemolysis or infection), and should be immediately referred.

If jaundice is marked over the next week, a heel prick test should be performed to assess the bilirubin concentration, as even physiological jaundice can cause encephalopathy if levels are too high.

Any jaundice that persists for over 10 days should be referred to exclude pathological causes (e.g. hypothyroidism, mild haemolysis, infection and liver disease, including biliary atresia).

Theme: Medication (analgesia) in a breastfeeding mother

(50) B and D

Discussion

Questions regarding drugs that are contraindicated during pregnancy and breastfeeding are relatively common. Consider especially medications that are used to treat chronic conditions such as epilepsy and asthma.

Paper 2 Questions

Theme: NICE guidelines for management of obesity

Options:

A   1
B   1.5
C.   2
D   2.5
E   3
F   3.5
G   4
H   4.5
I   5
J   6
K   7
L   8
M   9
N   10
O   11
P   12
Q   24
R   27
S   28
T   30
U   40
V   50

Please fit the correct numbers into the following sentences based on the NICE guidelines for obesity (December 2006).

People starting orlistat should meet the following criteria:

(1) BMI equal or greater than __ kg/m^2 with no comorbidity.

(2) BMI equal or greater than __ kg/m^2 in the presence of significant comorbidities (type II diabetes/hypertension/hyperlipidaemia).

(3) Continuation of therapy beyond __ months should be supported by evidence

(4) of a loss of __ % of body weight since initiating therapy.

(5) People starting sibutramine should have a BMI of equal or greater than __ kg/m^2 with obesity related risk factors.

(6) Treatment with sibutramine is not recommended beyond the licensed duration of __ months.

(7) Consider surgery for people with a BMI of __ kg/m^2 or more with no associated risk factors if all appropriate non-surgical measures have failed to

(8) achieve or maintain adequate clinically beneficial weight loss for at least __ months.

Theme: Audiograms

Options:

Choose the audiogram that best fits each of the following descriptions.

(9) A 54-year-old pneumatic drill operator has noticed that he is having difficulty hearing conversation on the telephone and in noisy environments.

(10) A 40-year-old woman says that her right ear feels blocked and sounds are muffled. On examination she has a lot of wax in that ear.

(11) A 76-year-old man is concerned that he is finding it difficult to hear words clearly because 'everyone mumbles nowadays'.

(12) A 24-year-old has severe bilateral deafness following meningitis as a child.

O = left ear   X = right ear

A
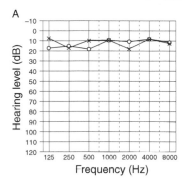

B
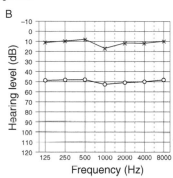

C
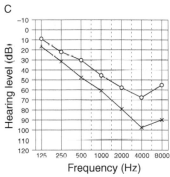

D
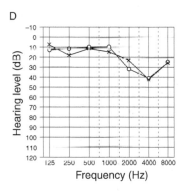

E
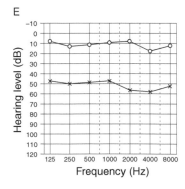

F
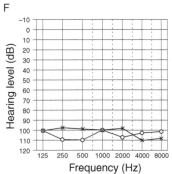

Theme: Childhood infections

Options:

A   Rubella
B   Measles
C   Fifth disease (parvovirus)
D   Hand, foot and mouth disease
E   Chickenpox
F   Roseala infantum
G   Scarlet fever

Choose the illness that corresponds most appropriately to the description below.

(13) Lesions are characteristically red macules that progress rapidly from papules to vesicles to pustules to crusts.

(14) Lesions begin as discrete erythematous macules and papules, which coalesce into areas of confluent erythema. Bluish-white macules 1 mm in diameter may develop on a background of erythematous oral mucosa; these are pathognomonic for this condition.

(15) The illness characteristically causes malar erythema followed by a reticular rash on the extremities and trunk.

(16) Rose-pink macular lesions are preceded by a high fever in an otherwise well child.

(17) The illness typically starts with the abrupt onset of fever, sore throat and headache, followed by a papular erythematous rash on the trunk and extremities. There is often circumoral pallor and erythema and prominence of the papillae on the surface of the tongue.

Theme: Medications which interact with warfarin

(18)   A 78-year-old man is on warfarin for atrial fibrillation. His INR control is erratic.

Which three of the following medications are likely to have contributed to this?

A   Glibenclamide
B   Lamotrigine
C   Insulin
D   Phenytoin
E   Erythromycin
F   Co-amoxiclav

Theme: Pre-conception counselling in an insulin-dependent diabetic

(19)   A 29-year-old type I (insulin-dependent) diabetic comes to the surgery to talk about starting a family.

Which two of the following must be discussed?

A   Decrease daily insulin dose
B   Good glycaemic control
C   Start an ACE inhibitor
D   Start folic acid
E   Switch to an oral hypoglycaemic

Theme: Change in bowel habit

Options:

A   Inflammatory bowel disease
B   Irritable bowel syndrome
C   Colorectal malignancy
D   Infective gastroenteritis
E   Coeliac disease
F   Hyperthroidism

What are the likely diagnoses for the following patient scenarios?

(20) An 18-year-old woman comes to see you with abdominal bloating and pain that are relieved by defaecation.

(21) A 25-year-old woman with diarrhoea and weight loss over the past few months mentions an intensely itchy rash on her elbows.

(22) A 38-year-old woman with recurrent bouts of dysuria and persistently negative urine cultures has also been complaining of lower abdominal pain associated with passing loose motions with mucus.

(23) A 65-year-old woman presents with general lethargy and increasing frequency of defaecation, often passing 'ribbony' motions.

(24) An 80-year-old man presents with a 1-week history of diarrhoea and crampy abdominal pains. His wife had similar symptoms, but he is concerned because her symptoms only lasted for a day or so.

Theme: Good Medical Practice guidelines

(25) Which of the following have not been highlighted by the GMC in the Good Medical Practice guidelines?

Choose three.

A   Make the care of your patient your first concern
B   Treat every patient politely and considerately
C   Consider the equity of treatment decisions with regard to the resources of the NHS
D   Respect patients' dignity and right to confidentiality
E   Listen to the patient's relatives and respect their views
F   Give patients information in a way they can understand
G   Respect the rights of patients to be informed of decisions about their care
H   Keep your professional knowledge and skills up to date
I   Recognise the limits of your professional competence
J   Be honest and open and act with integrity
K   Support patients in caring for themselves
L   Never discriminate unfairly against patients or colleagues
M   Act quickly to protect patients from risk if you have good reason to believe that you or a colleague may be putting patients at risk
N   Never abuse your patients' trust in you
O   Work with colleagues in the ways that best serve patients' interests

Theme: Psychiatric diagnoses

Options:

A Abnormal grief reaction
B Borderline personality disorder
C Dementia
D Depression
E Generalised anxiety disorder
F Normal grief reaction

Which of the above are the most likely diagnoses for the following patient scenarios?

26 A 65-year-old woman lost her husband one month ago. She initially coped well, but as the weeks go on she has begun to feel hopeless and apathetic. She has lost her sense of purpose, is becoming socially withdrawn, and feels that there is little prospect of improvement.

27 A 70-year-old woman lost her husband four years ago. Since the loss she repeatedly requests urgent home visits for very minor problems. On one of these visits you notice that her husband's coat is still on its hook and she seems to be talking to him when she goes into the kitchen to make a cup of tea.

28 An 88-year-old man lost his wife two years ago. He had been coping very well until his daughter moved to Spain for her retirement. Now he has no appetite, is not sleeping, wakes up in the middle of the night and has stopped attending the rotary club.

29 A 36-year-old woman lost her husband six weeks ago. She still feels his presence in the house and talks to him, often sensing that he responds to her. She finds it comforting to feel that he is still with her, but her parents are concerned that this is abnormal.

Theme: Shoulder problems

Options:

A   Rotator cuff injury
B   Adhesive capsulitis
C   Acromio-clavicular joint problem
D   Ruptured long head of biceps
E   Ruptured short head of biceps
F   Shoulder dislocation

What are the likely diagnoses for the following patients?

(30) A 50-year-old woman has a 2-week history of increasing pain and global restriction of movement in her shoulder.

(31) A 50-year-old woman has had many months of pain in the top of her shoulder, with limited abduction of the arm. Rotation is preserved.

(32) A 30-year-old body builder felt 'something give' when he was lifting weights the day before. Now he has discomfort on lifting his arm, but has retained full range of movement. There is a swelling in the upper arm on flexion of the elbow.

(33) A 50-year-old woman presents with several weeks of pain in the upper arm, which is usually worse at night. Examination reveals pain on abduction of the arm between 60 and 120 degrees.

Theme: Haematological malignancies

Options:

A   Acute lymphoblastic leukaemia
B   Acute myeloid leukaemia
C   Chronic lymphocytic leukaemia
D   Chronic myeloid leukaemia
E   Hodgkin's lymphoma
F   Non-Hodgkin's lymphoma
G   Burkitt's lymphoma
H   Polycythaemia rubra vera
I   Myelofibrosis
J   Myeloma
K   Waldenstrom's macroglobulinaemia
L   Hairy-cell leukaemia

Choose the most appropriate diagnoses for the following patient vignettes.

(34) A 70-year-old man presents with postural bone pain. He has a raised ESR, normal liver function, increased urea, creatinine and urate, and an M-band on serum electrophoresis.

(35) An elderly man presents with breathlessness and abdominal discomfort. Examination reveals gross hepatosplenomegaly, a full blood count shows low haemoglobin, and subsequent blood film shows tear-drop red blood cells.

(36) A 6-year-old Sudanese refugee presents with asymmetrical facial swelling. He has a positive monospot.

(37) A 45-year-old man presents with insidious weight loss. He has a dramatically raised white cell count, mild anaemia, and positive Philadelphia chromosome.

(38) A 3-year-old boy presents with severe pains in his legs, easy bruising and recurrent upper respiratory tract infections over the past couple of months. Full blood count reveals pancytopenia.

Theme: Travellers' infections

Options:

A   Amoebic dysentery
B   Giardiasis
C   Hookworm
D   Malaria
E   Typhoid
F   Rabies

Choose the infection that best fits each of the following clinical scenarios.

(39) A 31-year-old returned from a three week-trip to India ten days ago. He now has a two-day history of generally feeling unwell, with high fever, cough and constipation. He has noticed pinkish macules on his trunk.

(40) An 18-year-old student has been backpacking in Vietnam and returned six weeks ago. He is now suffering with intermittent headaches, malaise and anorexia interspersed with fevers, rigors and sweats.

(41) A 29-year-old woman has been on a canoeing holiday in South Africa. Within two weeks of her return she has had 'explosive diarrhoea' (she hasn't noticed any blood in it), but feels otherwise well.

Theme: Grading system used for symptoms of prostatism

(42) What grading system is commonly used for symptoms of prostatism?

A United Urology Questionnaire
B International Prostate Symptom Score
C Edinburgh Scale of Prostatism
D Alder Urinary Obstruction Score
E Scottish Prostatic Symptomatology Scoring System

Theme: Dermatology

Options:

A Pityriasis rosea
B Xerosis
C Acanthosis nigricans
D Granuloma annulare
E Melasma
F Psoriasis
G Lichen simplex
H Folliculitis
I Alopecia areata
J Furunculosis
K Tinea unguium
L Lichen planus
M Keratosis pilaris
N Hydradenitis suppurativa
O Kerion
P Tinea versicolor

Choose the most likely diagnosis for each scenario.

43. A 19-year-old student complains of itchy raised lesions on his wrists. He has a lacy white pattern inside his mouth.

44. A 16-year-old girl presents with rough skin on her upper arms. On close examination this is seen to consist of tiny papules in a grid-like distribution.

45. A 32-year-old man presents with a 2-year history of recurrent painful nodules and abscesses in his axillae.

46. An 11-year-old Afro-Caribbean has a boggy, pustular, indurated plaque on his scalp.

47. A 25-year-old man presents with a 6-month history of well-defined oval macules, that are pink/tan in colour, on his trunk, upper arms and neck.

Theme: Deaths reported to the coroner

48. Which two of the following deaths should be reported to the coroner?

A   A 76-year-old with mesothelioma who has previously worked with asbestos
B   Sudden death in a 48-year-old with multiple sclerosis
C   A 92-year-old who was visited by the GP ten days ago
D   A 76-year-old smoker with terminal COPD
E   Miscarriage at 14 weeks

Theme: Symptoms associated with vertigo

(49) In a patient presenting with vertigo, which one of the following associated symptoms gives most cause for concern?

A   Nausea
B   Nystagmus
C   Paroxysmal
D   Rapid onset
E   Tinnitus
F   Worse at night

Theme: Right of access to the medical records

(50) Which two of the following cases would have automatic right of access to the medical records they request?

A   The widow of a recently deceased patient would like a copy of his notes dating back 20 years or so to when he was diagnosed with hypertension

B   A very bright and articulate 14-year-old girl who has cystic fibrosis requests to see her records

C   A solicitor sends you a letter requesting a full copy of one of your patient's notes. There is a signed consent form enclosed

D   A mother requests access to her 15-year-old daughter's notes. The family are moving abroad and she would like to take them with her

Paper 2 Answers

Theme: NICE guidelines for management of obesity

1. T
2. S
3. E
4. I
5. R
6. P
7. U
8. J

Discussion

This is a topic which is likely to become more and more important because of the projected number of people suffering from the condition and the associated medical implications. The most recent NICE guidelines (www.nice.org.uk/guidance/CG43) stipulate quite strongly the criteria under which the drug treatments may be used and also when surgical referral is appropriate. Note that they have removed one of the original criteria from the guidelines which stated that the patient should have lost 3 kg in weight before they were eligible for a trial of orlistat. The guidelines also cover obesity in childhood and how waist circumference should be taken into account when assessing a person's risk.

Theme: Audiograms

⑨ D

⑩ E

⑪ C

⑫ F

Discussion

You may be asked to interpret audiograms in the exam. This audiogram shows the normal speech sounds.

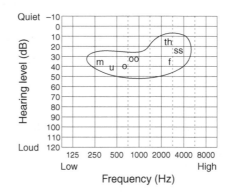

The quietest sounds are highest up on the graph. In the above examples, 'A' is a normal audiogram. The higher-frequency sounds such as ss, th and f are to the right of the graph. 'E' shows a typical conductive deafness audiogram. 'C' shows an audiogram of presbycusis (age-related sensorineural deafness). 'F' is a severe bilateral deafness.

Theme: Childhood infections

⑬ E

⑭ B

⑮ C

⑯ F

⑰ G

Discussion

This set of questions is very wordy, but cutting through this, the individual questions are not difficult. Koplik spots and strawberry tongue have deliberately been described rather than named to ensure that the candidate knows what these conditions actually look like. The question also highlights the importance of understanding dermatological terminology.

Theme: Medications which interact with warfarin

⑱   A D and E

Discussion

There will be some pharmacotherapeutic questions, so it is worth looking at the common interactions. However, in reality you will have a *BNF* and a question like this is only worth one mark, so don't worry too much if you are unsure.

Theme: Pre-conception counselling in an insulin-dependent diabetic

(19) B and D

Pre-pregnancy counselling should include the necessity for strict blood glucose control and folic acid supplementation. ACE inhibitors, statins and oral hypoglycaemics are contraindicated in pregnancy.

Insulin requirements usually increase rather than decrease in pregnancy.

Theme: Change in bowel habit

(20) B
(21) E
(22) B
(23) C
(24) D

Discussion

Irritable bowel syndrome is extremely common, but if it first presents over the age of 40 years, malignancy needs to be excluded (especially if the patient is lethargic – is she anaemic?). Irritable bowel syndrome will often be presented with other 'functional' disorders such as non-ulcer dyspepsia, disproportionate breathlessness and, in this example, functional cystitis.

Theme: Good Medical Practice guidelines

(25) C G and E

Discussion

The GMC website, www.gmc-uk.org/guidance, has the correct list of these 'duties' as well as other ethical information. Note that there is no mention of justice in terms of treatment provision or any consideration of NHS limitations. There is no mention of relatives, and patients should be involved in decision making rather than informed of it.

Theme: Psychiatric diagnoses

(26) F

(27) A

(28) D

(29) F

Discussion

There is a thin line between 'normal' and 'abnormal' grief. The defined stages of grieving are as follows.

1   The immediate effects of bereavement are characterised by disbelief and numbness, and last for days or weeks. The acute effects of grief are often positive symptoms such as crying out, searching and agitation.

2   The intermediate stage of grief is characterised by negative symptoms such as depression, despair and apathy.

3   Resolution of the grief and reinvestment of emotional energies should have occurred within 2 years of the loss.

Grief is considered abnormal if it is delayed, prolonged or exhibits features such as hypochondriasis, alcohol or drug abuse, or affective symptoms.

Theme: Shoulder problems

(30) B

(31) C

(32) D

(33) A

Discussion

This question could also be asked as a management question, for which the answer in most cases would be NSAID/physiotherapy. There are different possible injuries to the rotator cuff. Acute and chronic tendinitis will usually settle eventually, but if a significant tear is suspected (pain improves but active abduction is limited to 45–60 degrees, with full passive abduction) in a young active person, they should be considered for surgical repair.

Theme: Haematological malignancies

(34) J

(35) I

(36) G

(37) D

(38) A

Discussion

Don't panic! Questions like this will come up, but they are few and far between. This is an example of a question where the time and effort involved in learning this level of information have to be balanced against the number of marks you will earn for it and the likelihood of the question appearing at all.

Theme: Travellers' infections

(39) E

(40) D

(41) B

Discussion

An awareness of some of the diseases that travellers can acquire is important.

Malaria should always be excluded. Typhoid is caused by *Salmonella typhi* and can cause rose spots on the trunk, although these are not always seen.

Theme: Grading system used for symptoms of prostatism

(42) B

Discussion

The International Prostate Symptom Score (IPSS) is a series of questions, devised by the American Urological Association, that grades prostatic symptoms over the last month. It is useful for monitoring symptoms over time and also for providing a guide as to when to refer.

Theme: Dermatology

(43) L
(44) M
(45) N
(46) O
(47) P

Discussion

Dermatological conditions are a favourite question and are likely to come up. Make sure that you know the difference between the various rashes, many of which have similar-sounding names. In Question 47, the history is too long to be pityriasis versicolor.

Theme: Deaths reported to the coroner

(48) A and B

Discussion

Deaths which must be reported to the coroner include the following:

- any death which was sudden, unexplained, uncertified by a medical practitioner or surrounded by suspicious circumstances
- any death that may be due to an industrial injury or disease, or to accident, violence, neglect or poisoning (excluding alcoholism)

- any death that occurred during an operation or before recovery from the effect of an anaesthetic
- any death where the deceased had not been treated by a doctor during their illness
- any death where the doctor attending the deceased did not see them within 14 days before or after death
- any death that occurred in police custody or in prison
- stillbirths and terminations of pregnancy.

Theme: Symptoms associated with vertigo

 B

Discussion

Vertigo associated with nystagmus or any other neurological symptom is a red flag, suggesting an underlying central nervous system lesion (e.g. cerebellar tumour or multiple sclerosis).

Vertigo is a common problem and the differential diagnosis should be known, including labyrinthine conditions, Ménière's disease, benign positional vertigo and vertebro-basilar ischaemia.

Theme: Right of access to the medical records

(50) B and C

Discussion

There are three acts that you should be aware of:

- the Data Protection Act
- the Access to Health Records Act
- the Access to Medical Reports Act.

Further information about these is available on the GMC and BMA websites, www.gmc-uk.org and www.bma.org.uk.

There is no statutory right of access to deceased people's notes dating back before 1991, and there should only be access to information which is relevant to any claim that the third party may be making.

Competent patients have right of access to their records. This includes competent minors, and if the parents want access they must apply for it. A competent person can give consent for a third party to have access to their records.

Paper 3 Questions

Theme: NICE guidelines for the management of heart failure

Options:

A   Full blood count
B   Urea and electrolytes
C   Liver function tests
D   Thyroid function tests
E   Natriuretic peptide
F   Electrocardiogram
G   Chest X-ray
H   Spirometry
I   Trans-thoracic echocardiogram
J   Trans-oesophageal echocardiogram
K   Radionucleotide cardiac imaging
L   Cardiac magnetic resonance imaging

Please fill in the gaps below.

The NICE guidelines for the management of heart failure suggest that all diagnoses should be reviewed and all patients should have an ① and a ② where available. If both of these tests are normal, heart failure is unlikely and an alternative diagnosis should be considered and tested for by blood tests, ③, urinalysis and peak flow or ④.

If one or more of the initial tests are abnormal, a ⑤ should be performed. If this confirms cardiac failure, treatment should be instigated.

Theme: Free prescriptions

⑥   Which two of the following conditions or circumstances are not entitled to free prescriptions?

A   Epilepsy
B   Patient with colostomy
C   Woman who gave birth 10 months ago
D   Chronic glaucoma
E   Employed 62-year-old
F   Diet-controlled diabetic
G   Hypoparathyroidism

Theme: Epilepsy medication monitoring

Options:

A   Liver function
B   Plasma drug concentration
C   Serum potassium
D   Thyroid function
E   Visual fields

For each of the anti-epilepsy medications below, choose the appropriate monitoring that should be performed.

⑦   Phenytoin.

⑧   Sodium valproate.

⑨   Vigabatrin.

Theme: Prostate cancer

(10) Which of the following statements about prostate cancer is incorrect?

A   A raised PSA is not diagnostic of prostate cancer
B   Prostate cancer is the second most common cause of cancer death in men
C   PSA screening fulfils Wilson's screening criteria
D   Prostate cancer is rare in men under the age of 50 years
E   A raised PSA can be caused by prostatitis or urinary infection

Theme: Antipsychotic medication

Options:

A   Oral atypical antipsychotics
B   Depot risperidone
C   Depot haloperidol
D   Oral typical antipsychotic
E   Clozapine

What would be the appropriate choice of medication for the following patients?

(11) A 24-year-old man has been having florid delusions and hallucinations, and is thought disordered. He believes that his thoughts are being broadcast on the radio. This is his first episode, there is no history of drug abuse, and physical assessment is normal.

(12) A 36-year-old schizophrenic has been deteriorating over the preceding 6 months. He was given olanzapine for a couple of months and was then tried on haloperidol for a couple of months by the early diagnosis in psychosis team. Despite this,

he is becoming more withdrawn, exhibiting strange behaviour within the supportive home where he lives, and he believes that the IRA controls his thoughts.

(13) A 46-year-old man with a diagnosis of schizophrenia has been receiving depot haloperidol for several years. He comes regularly to the surgery to have his injection, is managing to hold down a job with the Post Office, and feels well in himself.

(14) A 40-year-old woman with recurrent psychotic episodes has become quite thought disordered and chaotic over the past week. She has tried various antipsychotics in the past, and has suffered minor dyskinesias as a result of the ones she used many years ago.

Theme: Constipation

Options:

A   Lactulose
B   Co-danthramer
C   Senokot
D   Glycerine suppository
E   Micralax enema
F   Fybogel
G   Castor oil

What would be the most appropriate choice of laxative for each of the following patients?

(15) A 30-year-old woman has not opened her bowels since a particularly traumatic vaginal delivery a week ago. She has tried prune juice and Fybogel.

(16) A 70-year-old man has had lifelong bowel difficulties. He has used castor oil in the past with great success, and is due to go away for a few weeks. He asks your advice as to what he should take with him, as he always becomes constipated when he is away from home.

(17) An elderly woman has been taking lactulose and Senokot for a couple of weeks. She has become really uncomfortable and would like something stronger.

(18) A 3-year-old boy has had difficulties going to the toilet after passing a hard motion a couple of weeks ago causing a small anal tear. He has been drinking more and taking lactulose twice daily, but is still having difficulty.

(19) A 60-year-old with an advanced metastatic malignancy has been on lactulose and Senokot to counteract his morphine, but they do not seem to be working very well.

Theme: Meta-analysis

Options:

A	1.00
B	1.50
C	1.26
D	3.00
E	0.50
F	2.50
G	2.00
H	6.25
I	0.99
J	1.99
K	3.00
L	4.00

Choose the correct answer for each of the following questions.

(20) How many of these studies show a significant reduction in duration of symptoms and are applicable to a 24-year-old man with irritable bowel syndrome who presents with a 2-day history of suspected influenza?

(21) How many studies demonstrate no significant reduction in duration of symptoms when comparing treatment with zanamivir to placebo in an otherwise healthy population?

(22) What is the average reduction in symptom duration in a high-risk patient (in days)?

(23) What is the average reduction in symptom duration compared with placebo in the most highly weighted trial of the high-risk group (in days)?

(24) What is the average reduction in duration of symptoms in a patient who is otherwise healthy (in days)?

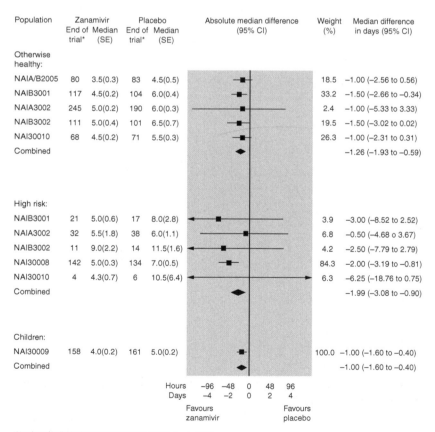

Population	Zanamivir End of trial*	Median (SE)	Placebo End of trial*	Median (SE)	Absolute median difference (95% CI)	Weight (%)	Median difference in days (95% CI)
Otherwise healthy:							
NAIA/B2005	80	3.5(0.3)	83	4.5(0.5)		18.5	−1.00 (−2.56 to 0.56)
NAIB3001	117	4.5(0.2)	104	6.0(0.4)		33.2	−1.50 (−2.66 to −0.34)
NAIA3002	245	5.0(0.2)	190	6.0(0.3)		2.4	−1.00 (−5.33 to 3.33)
NAIB3002	111	5.0(0.4)	101	6.5(0.7)		19.5	−1.50 (−3.02 to 0.02)
NAI30010	68	4.5(0.2)	71	5.5(0.3)		26.3	−1.00 (−2.31 to 0.31)
Combined							−1.26 (−1.93 to −0.59)
High risk:							
NAIB3001	21	5.0(0.6)	17	8.0(2.8)		3.9	−3.00 (−8.52 to 2.52)
NAIA3002	32	5.5(1.8)	38	6.0(1.1)		6.8	−0.50 (−4.68 to 3.67)
NAIB3002	11	9.0(2.2)	14	11.5(1.6)		4.2	−2.50 (−7.79 to 2.79)
NAI30008	142	5.0(0.3)	134	7.0(0.5)		84.3	−2.00 (−3.19 to −0.81)
NAI30010	4	4.3(0.7)	6	10.5(6.4)		6.3	−6.25 (−18.76 to 0.75)
Combined							−1.99 (−3.08 to −0.90)
Children:							
NAI30009	158	4.0(0.2)	161	5.0(0.2)		100.0	−1.00 (−1.60 to −0.40)
Combined							−1.00 (−1.60 to −0.40)

Hours −96 −48 0 48 96
Days   −4   −2 0 2   4
Favours zanamivir   Favours placebo

*Number of individuals with symptoms alleviated at end of trial.

Theme: Interpreting blood test results

Options:

A   Chronic renal failure
B   Dehydration
C   Familial benign hypercalcaemia
D   Malignancy
E   Milk-alkali syndrome
F   Primary hyperparathyroidism
G   Primary hypoparathyroidism
H   Sarcoidosis
I   Vitamin D treatment

Reference ranges:

Sodium	135–145
Potassium	3.5–5
Urea	2.5–6.7
Creatinine	70–140
Hb	13.5–18
WCC	4–11
Platelets	150–400
Corrected calcium	2.12–2.65
Phosphate	0.8–1.45
Albumin	35–50
Total protein	60–80
Alanine aminotransferase (ALT)	5–35
Alkaline phosphatase	30–150
Bilirubin	3–17

What are the likely causes of the following patients' symptoms and/ or blood test results?

(25) A diabetic patient has been feeling progressively more tired and lethargic over the past few months. Blood tests show the following:

Sodium	135
Potassium	4.9
Urea	20
Creatinine	235
Hb	10.4
WCC	6.2
Platelets	180
Corrected calcium	2.12
Phosphate	1.54
Albumin	35
Total protein	65
ALT	40
Alkaline phosphatase	165
Bilirubin	12

(26) A 64-year-old woman complains of feeling generally unwell for several months with aches and pains, poor appetite, nausea and a low mood. She has been vomiting profusely over the past couple of days. Blood tests show the following:

Sodium	140
Potassium	4.5
Urea	14
Creatinine	145
Hb	13
WCC	7
Platelets	200
Corrected calcium	3
Phosphate	0.77
Albumin	40
Total protein	70
ALT	40
Alkaline phosphatase	160
Bilirubin	14

(27) Routine blood tests of a 45-year-old man reveal mildly raised calcium levels but nothing else. He mentions that both his sister and his mother have also been told that they have high calcium levels.

Theme: Elbow, wrist and hand problems

Options:

A Carpal tunnel syndrome
B Dislocated elbow
C Ganglion
D Lateral epicondylitis
E Medial epicondylitis
F Olecranon bursitis
G Osteoarthritis
H Pulled elbow
I Repetitive strain injury
J Tenosynovitis
K Trigger finger

What is the likely problem for each of the following patients?

(28) A 65-year-old man presents with pain in the wrist that is made worse by gardening for prolonged periods. On examination there is pain over the radial styloid on adducting and flexing his thumb.

(29) A 58-year-old office worker has pain and swelling in the elbow. You manage to aspirate some fluid, which has a negative Gram stain and no crystals.

(30) A 55-year-old man has pain in his elbow that has been building up over the past few weeks. It is particularly noticeable on resisted pronation of the wrist.

(31) A 46-year-old woman has pain in the lateral 3½ digits with some pins and needles. On examination there is some wasting of the thenar eminence.

(32) A 20-year-old woman has a smooth, firm, painless swelling on her wrist.

Theme: Eligibility for treatment

(33) Which two of the following cases would be liable to a charge for the treatment they have received/are receiving?

A   A refugee patient is awaiting news as to whether he has been awarded leave to stay. He is HIV positive and due to commence antiretroviral therapy

B   A 66-year-old English man has retired to Florida, having worked in the UK for 45 years. He comes back after 6 months to visit his daughter and get his annual blood tests and a repeat prescription for his statin

C   An Iranian diabetic man has come to the UK to visit his family for a couple of months. He has renal failure for which he receives dialysis in Iran, and his daughter has brought him to see you to arrange admission for dialysis and ongoing care while he is here

D   A 24-year-old French man who is at university in the UK presents with symptoms suggestive of renal colic. He is referred to the hospital and subsequently requires surgical extraction of the stone

Theme: Blocked nose

Options:

A Adenoidal hypertrophy
B Allergic rhinitis
C Carcinoma
D Foreign body
E Nasal polyps
F Nasal septal deviation
G Papilloma
H Rhinitis medicamentosa
I   Septal haematoma
J   Unilateral choanal atresia
K Vasomotor rhinitis

Which is the most likely diagnosis for each of the following?

(34) A 3-year-old with a unilateral foul-smelling bloody discharge.

(35) A 19-year-old rugby player who has been hit on the nose and is now complaining of bilateral nasal obstruction. On examination there is a bright red midline swelling visible from both nostrils.

(36) A 43-year-old is suffering from chronic nasal obstruction and discharge. She has used over-the-counter nasal sprays for months and feels that the problem is worsening.

(37) A 78-year-old has noticed right-sided nasal obstruction associated with a bloody discharge that has developed over the last month.

(38) A 22-year-old complains that the same time every year she develops a blocked nose with profuse watery discharge.

Theme: Failure to thrive

Options:

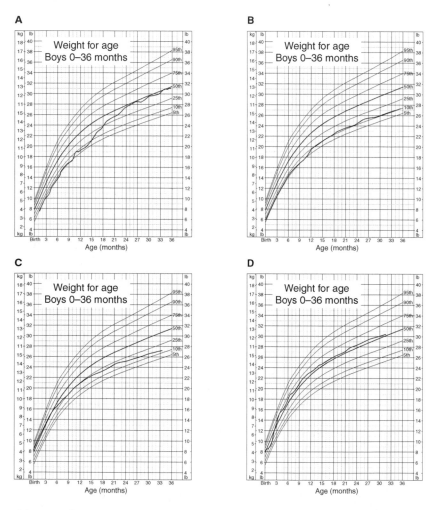

A Weight for age Boys 0–36 months

B Weight for age Boys 0–36 months

C Weight for age Boys 0–36 months

D Weight for age Boys 0–36 months

Choose the growth chart that best fits each of the clinical scenarios below.

(39) Both of this boy's parents are on the 5th centile for height.

(40) This child is living in a chaotic family environment. Their mother is a drug abuser.

(41) This child was born with congenital heart disease. This has now been operated on to reverse the defect.

(42) Uncomplicated birth and infancy.

(43) This child's mother has been abusing drugs and alcohol. His grandmother is now looking after him.

Theme: Yellow card reporting system

(44) Which one of the following statements about the yellow card reporting system is incorrect?

A Yellow cards can be found in the back of the *BNF*
B All suspected adverse drug effects should be reported for black triangle drugs
C The yellow card reporting system is one of the circumstances in which breaching patient confidentiality may be justified
D It includes the use of over-the-counter medications
E Only serious adverse effects should be reported for established drugs and vaccines
F The black triangle remains with a drug for 5 years after its introduction

Theme: Hormone replacement therapy

(45) Which of the following statements about hormone replacement therapy is correct?

A It decreases the risk of cardiovascular disease
B Tibolone does not increase the risk of breast cancer
C It decreases the risk of gall-bladder disease
D It can increase the risk of breast cancer after only one or two years of use
E It is recommended as first-line treatment for preventing osteoporosis

Theme: Skin lesions

Options:

A Angioma
B Seborrhoeic wart
C Melanoma
D Comedone
E Bowen's disease
F Viral wart
G Lipoma
H Keratoacanthoma
I Basal-cell carcinoma
J Sebaceous cyst
K Dermatofibroma

Choose the diagnosis that is most likely for each of the lesions shown below.

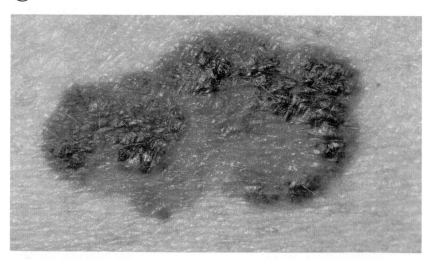

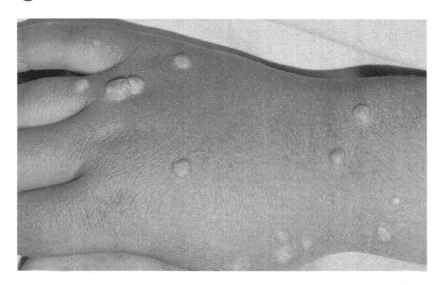

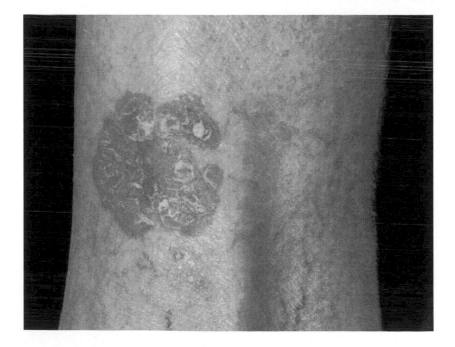

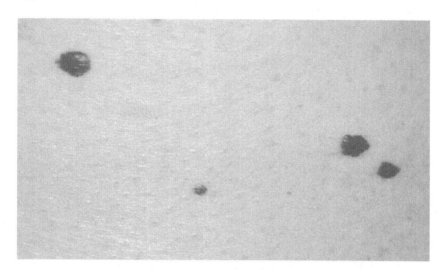

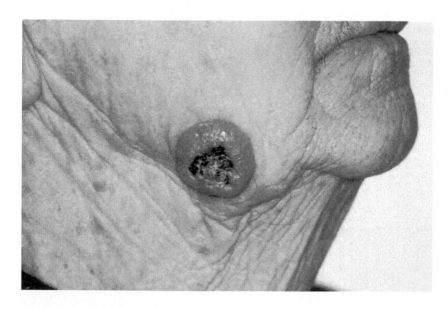

Paper 3 Answers

Theme: NICE guidelines for the management of heart failure

1. F
2. E
3. G
4. H
5. I

Discussion

See the NICE guidelines at www.nice.org.uk/pdf/Full_HF_Guideline.pdf. You need to be relatively well versed in the recently published guidelines affecting general practice. It is probably a good idea to concentrate particularly on the ones that are being flagged up in the contract. An alternative question for heart failure would be to go through the treatment algorithm.

From the point of view of technique, look at the grammar in order to get the correct answer into its respective gap (for example, look at 'a' vs. 'an').

Theme: Free prescriptions

6. D and F

Discussion

Note the negative in the question. A general rule is that free prescriptions are available for any deficiency (e.g. hypopituitarism, hypoadrenalism or hypothyroidism). Any diabetic except those controlled by diet alone, and patients with epilepsy and permanent fistulas are the other clinical conditions. Non-clinical circumstances include children under 16 years of age, or under 19 years in full-time education, adults over 60 years, pregnant women or those who have given birth in the last 12 months, and anyone who is receiving benefits.

Theme: Epilepsy medication monitoring

(7) B

(8) A

(9) E

Discussion

Due to the narrow therapeutic index of phenytoin, plasma drug levels should be measured regularly until optimum dosing is achieved. Plasma drug levels are also useful for determining optimum dosage with carbamazepine, ethosuxamide and phenobarbitone.

Liver toxicity has been reported with the use of sodium valproate, so the advice in the *BNF* is to monitor liver function before therapy and during the first 6 months of therapy.

Vigabatrin is associated with visual-field defects, which can occur from one month to several years after starting treatment. The manufacturer's advice is to test visual fields before treatment and at 6-month intervals during treatment.

Theme: Prostate cancer

(10) C

Discussion

It is worth revising the pros and cons of prostate screening, as it could come up in the essay paper.

PSA screening does not fulfil Wilson's screening criteria as it is not sensitive or specific, there is no consensus on how it should be treated, and the natural history is not well known, as it can be either asymptomatic and slow growing or fast and aggressive, but there is no way of predicting the type.

Further details can be found at www.doh.gov.uk/nsc/pdfs/prostate_cancer.pdf

Theme: Antipsychotic medication

(11) A
(12) E
(13) C
(14) A

Discussion

NICE guidelines on the management of psychosis and the use of antipsychotic medication were released in 2002. They are summarised at www.gpnotebook.co.uk and www.nice.org.uk. They do suggest greater GP input, especially with regard to early diagnosis and initiation of therapy.

Depot risperidone is fairly new and supposedly set to revolutionise the management of chronic schizophrenia. The early diagnosis in psychosis teams are becoming ubiquitous, and are keen to get their hands on people to reduce chronic morbidity. You would be very unlikely to have much to do with the prescribing of a drug such as clozapine, but it is worth knowing the indication and the potential harm that it may cause in case you are asked to be involved in the prescribing of this drug.

The patient in Question 12 would need to be involved in a discussion of the potential long-term side-effects of the 'typical' depot antipsychotic, but if he were well maintained and happy on it, then it would be appropriate to continue.

Theme: Constipation

(15) A
(16) G
(17) D
(18) C
(19) B

Discussion

Easy marks? They always seem to sneak in a question about senna postnatally, as it causes quite nasty diarrhoea in the breastfed infant. The 70-year-old has had success with castor oil for many years, and if away from home should stick to what he knows. The elderly woman could try an enema, but this would probably involve a district nurse, so to save them a job try the glycerine suppository first.

Theme: Meta-analysis

(20) A
(21) L
(22) J

㉓ G

㉔ C

Discussion

There will be questions asking you to interpret charts like these in the essay paper. In the EMQ paper, expect to have to dissect the data a little. You should be able to score full marks with a bit of concentration!

The key concept in this question is that of significance. If a confidence interval crosses zero, it is not a significant result. In terms of trial weighting, a narrow confidence interval suggests a more impressive result.

Theme: Interpreting blood test results

㉕ A

㉖ F

㉗ C

Discussion

Diabetes is the commonest cause of renal impairment and subsequent renal failure. Remember that the kidneys manufacture erythropoietin – hence the anaemia seen in chronic renal failure. Urate levels rise in parallel with plasma urea, and high levels are not diagnostic of primary hyperuricaemia. Plasma phosphate levels tend to rise and calcium levels fall. There may be a secondary hyperparathyroidism, which leads to increased alkaline phosphatase activity.

Hyperparathyroidism will cause a normal/low phosphate level, whereas malignancies will tend to cause a normal/raised phosphate level, and bony metastases in particular will increase the alkaline phosphatase very significantly. Primary hyperparathyroidism can cause raised alkaline phosphatase as a late manifestation, as the PTH stimulates osteoclasts to liberate calcium, which in turn causes a secondary osteoblastic reaction (these manufacture alkaline phosphatase). There would usually be a raised urea level with a malignant hypercalcaemia. There will often be a hypercalcaemia related to malignancies, such as is seen in non-small-cell cancers of the lung, which can cause secretion of PTH-related peptide.

Familial hypercalcaemia is common, benign, and requires no treatment.

Theme: Elbow, wrist and hand problems

(28) J

(29) F

(30) E

(31) A

(32) C

Discussion

Retirement and gardening seem to bring on many problems for people! This is also known as de Quervain's synovitis. The differential would be osteoarthritis, which also typically affects the first carpometacarpal joint, causing pain at the base of the thumb.

Bursitis can be extremely painful, and is generally fairly acute and caused by repeated pressure on the elbow (e.g. during office work).

Lateral epicondylitis (tennis elbow) pain is reproduced by forced extension of the wrist. Medial epicondylitis (golfer's elbow) pain is reproduced by resisted pronation of the wrist. The pain is also reproduced by pressure over the insertion of the tendon into the respective epicondyle.

Carpal tunnel syndrome due to compression of the median nerve is associated with arthritis, hypothyroidism, pregnancy and obesity, but is often idiopathic. Remember phalens (**PH**lexion of wrist) and tinnels (**T**apping over flexor retinaculum).

Theme: Eligibility for treatment

(33) B and C

Discussion

There are rules as to who is entitled to receive medical care courtesy of the NHS, although their implementation is not always so regimented.

Anyone considered to be resident in the UK is entitled to free treatment, and this can be from the moment the plane lands. However, if they intend to stay for less than 6 months, they are not considered to be resident. UK nationals who live abroad for 3 months or more are no longer considered to be resident, even if they are paying tax and National Insurance.

People from the European Economic Area (if carrying the correct forms) and refugees (regardless of status) are entitled to standard NHS care.

Emergency care and immediately necessary treatment (for up to 14 days) are provided to all, as is compulsory psychiatric treatment and communicable disease treatment (except for HIV, which can be tested for but not treated).

More information is available at www.doh.gov.uk/overseas visitors/index.htm.

Theme: Blocked nose

(34) D
(35) I

(36) H

(37) C

(38) B

Discussion

Blocked nose is a common general practice problem, and the causes can be diverse.

Unilateral nasal obstruction in the elderly is considered to be carcinoma until proved otherwise, although polyps are a possible cause. Ambiguity can arise in this kind of question, as it could be argued that polyps are more likely, but ask yourself what the underlying aim of the question is. In this case it is to determine whether the candidate knows never to assume that unilateral nasal obstruction is benign in an elderly person, in which case it is better to opt for the answer that fulfils that criterion.

Rhinitis medicamentosa occurs as a result of overuse of the vasoconstricting decongestants, and there is a rebound worsening of the symptoms on discontinuing the medication.

A septal haematoma must be looked for in any case of nasal trauma, and needs evacuation if it is present, as it can cause septal cartilage necrosis and infection.

Theme: Failure to thrive

(39) B

(40) C

(41) A

(42) D

(43) A

Discussion

A   Low birth weight then normalises as conditions change.
B   Remains on the same centile even though it is below average.
C   Starts as normal birth weight and then falls across two centiles.
D   Normal fall-off around birth and then back to birth weight centile.

Failure to thrive is defined as weight consistently below the 3rd centile, or a progressive fall in growth either to the 3rd centile or based on the previous plotted growth curve.

- Causes can be categorised as organic or non-organic. Examples of organic conditions include systemic conditions (diabetes mellitus, respiratory or cardiac disease), chronic infection (TB) or gastro-intestinal problems (coeliac disease or chronic diarrhoea).
- Examples of non-organic conditions include malnutrition secondary to neglect or famine, and emotional problems.

Theme: Yellow card reporting system

 F

Discussion

There is no standard length of time for a drug to have a black triangle. It is usually reviewed after two years of availability.

Black triangles identify new drugs that are being intensely monitored by the Committee on Safety of Medicines (CSM) and the Medical and Healthcare Products Regulatory Agency (MHRA).

Black-triangle drugs should have all reactions reported, whether they are minor or serious. Established drugs only need to have serious reactions reported.

Theme: Hormone replacement therapy

 D

Discussion

The Million Women Study (Breast cancer and hormone replacement therapy in the Million Women Study. *Lancet* 2003; **362**: 419) has reinforced much of the information obtained in the Women's Health Initiative study published in the *Journal of the American Medical Association* in 2002.

The latest figures on breast cancer show that the relative risk of contracting the disease is as follows:

Combined HRT	RR	2.0
Oestrogen only	RR	1.3
Tibolone	RR	1.45

It is also confirmed that HRT does not offer cardiovascular benefit as was once thought, and that due to the risks involved it is now not recommended as first-line treatment for prophylaxis of osteoporosis.

It is important to know the current recommendations, as this topic comes up frequently both in this paper and in the essay paper.

Government recommendations can be found at www.mhra. gov.uk/

Theme: Skin lesions

- (46) C
- (47) F
- (48) E
- (49) A
- (50) H

Discussion

Photographs of dermatological lesions are regularly encountered in the nMRCGP® exam. Refresh your memory about the commoner lesions that are easily recognisable.

Paper 4 Questions

Theme: Haematology

Options:

A   Iron-deficiency anaemia
B   Anaemia of chronic disease
C   Vitamin B_{12} deficiency
D   Folate deficiency
E   Thalassaemia trait
F   Haemolysis
G   Aplastic anaemia

Reference ranges:

Haemoglobin	13.5–18 (men), 11.5–16 (women) g/dl
MCV	76–97 fl
Reticulocytes	$25–100 \times 10^9/l$
WCC	$4–11 \times 10^9/l$
Platelets	$150–400 \times 10^9/l$
Ferritin	12–200 µg/l
Vitamin B_{12}	0.13–0.68 nmol/l
Folate	0.36–1.44 µmol/l

What are the likely causes of the following blood test results?

(1) A 34-year-old Chinese man has a routine full blood count as part of an insurance medical.

Haemoglobin	11.5
MCV	74
Reticulocytes	50
WCC	6
Platelets	150
Ferritin	150
Vitamin B_{12}	0.5
Folate	1

(2) At a postnatal check the mother admits to feeling very tired.

Haemoglobin	10
MCV	74
Reticulocytes	110
WCC	8
Platelets	370
Ferritin	5
Vitamin B_{12}	0.15
Folate	0.45

(3) A 30-year-old woman has been feeling extremely tired and breathless on exertion over the past 2–3 weeks.

Haemoglobin	7
MCV	70
Reticulocytes	4
WCC	1
Platelets	20
Ferritin	150
Vitamin B_{12}	0.4
Folate	1.0

④ A 35-year-old epileptic patient has been fit-free on phenytoin for many years, and for this reason rarely attends for review.

Haemoglobin	12.5
MCV	105
Reticulocytes	80
WCC	6
Platelets	200
Ferritin	180
Vitamin B_{12}	0.4
Folate	0.2

Theme: Employment law

Options:

A 2 weeks
B 4 weeks
C 3 months
D 6 months
E 1 year
F 2 years
G 4 years

What is the correct time frame for each of the following situations?

⑤ Time in employment within which a written contract must be provided.

⑥ Period of employment after which an agreed period of notice should be given.

⑦ Length of notice required for planned maternity leave.

⑧ Duration of employment after which employees are entitled to redundancy pay.

Theme: Mouth problems

Options:

A   Aphthous ulcer
B   Leukoplakia
C   Mucocoele
D   Gingivitis
E   Oral candidiasis
F   Lichen planus
G   Basal-cell carcinoma
H   Angular stomatitis
I   Ulcerative stomatitis
J   Epithelioma
K   Leukaemia

What is the likely diagnosis for each of the following patients?

(9) A 45-year-old man is referred to you by his dental hygienist, who noticed pale grey opaque areas interspersed with a few red inflamed patches on his tongue while scraping the tobacco stains off his teeth.

(10) An elderly man with ill-fitting dentures complains of painful inflamed cracks at the corners of his mouth.

(11) The above patient also has a fissure on his lip that fails to respond to treatment, although the inflamed cracks at the corners of his mouth heal well.

(12) A 55-year-old man presents with bleeding gums. On examination there is a line of inflammation at the border of the gum, the interdental papillae are swollen, and he has halitosis.

(13) A 67-year-old man with COPD has recently had an infective exacerbation. He complains of an unpleasant taste in his mouth, and examination reveals white deposits adhering to the mucous membranes.

Theme: Bone problems

Options:

A   Bone tumour
B   Myeloma
C   Osteomalacia
D   Osteomyelitis
E   Osteoporosis
F   Paget's disease
G   Primary hyperparathyroidism
H   Rickets
I   Septic arthritis

What is the likely diagnosis for each of the following patients?

(14) An elderly man presents with a history of several months of dull aching bone pain that is made worse by exercise. On examination there is some bowing of the tibia. He has raised alkaline phosphatase but normal calcium, phosphate and PTH levels.

(15) A 67-year-old diabetic woman has a deep venous ulcer that is persistently infected despite several courses of oral antibiotics.

(16) A 63-year-old Afghanistani woman comes to see you with a proximal myopathy and general bone pains. Her calcium and phosphate levels are slightly low and her alkaline phosphatase level is raised.

(17) A 64-year-old woman presents with bone aches and pains, weight loss and fatigue. Blood tests reveal a mild anaemia, elevated urea and creatinine levels, raised serum calcium with low alkaline phosphatase levels, and a raised ESR.

Theme: Hip problems

Options:

A   Avascular necrosis
B   Fascia lata syndrome
C   Hip dislocation
D   Hip fracture
E   Hip infection
F   Malignancy
G   Meralgia paraesthetica
H   Osteoarthritis
I   Trochanteric bursitis

What is the likely diagnosis for each of the following patients?

(18) A 68-year-old man had a hip replacement 4 weeks ago having fractured his hip in a fall. He presents with a 10-day history of feeling unwell, intermittent fevers, weight loss and pain in the hip.

(19) A 72-year-old man presents with severe unremitting hip pain that has been becoming progressively worse over the past few weeks. He has lost some weight and also complains of prostatic symptoms.

(20) A 65-year-old woman presents with fairly acute pain over her greater trochanter. She has mild chronic osteoarthritis in both knees and hips.

(21) A 28-year-old man with sickle-cell disease presents with hip pain and is walking with a slight limp.

Theme: Interpretation of trial data

Options:

A   1/12
B   11/275
C   12/275
D   12/263
E   263/275
F   1/275
G   1/274
H   11/550
I   1
J   2
K   3
L   4
M   11
N   12
O   15
P   25
Q   250

There is a flu epidemic coming. The manager of a local residential home wonders whether her 25 residents should have oral prophylaxis in addition to influenza vaccination. The results of a recent study on influenza prophylaxis in a residential home setting are as follows:

Number of subjects   550
Number vaccinated   80
Number receiving influenza prophylaxis 275
Number receiving placebo   275
Duration of treatment   6 weeks
Number of influenza cases in treatment group
   1
Number of influenza cases in placebo group
  12

Answer the following questions with reference to the above data.

(22)   What is the risk of developing influenza without prophylaxis?

(23)   What is the percentage relative risk reduction for developing influenza when given prophylaxis?

(24)   What is the absolute risk reduction?

(25)   What is the number needed to treat?

Theme: Psychiatric disorders of childhood

Options:

A   Childhood schizophrenia
B   Separation anxiety disorder
C   Conduct disorder
D   Attention deficit hyperactivity disorder (ADHD)
E   Childhood depression
F   School refusal
G   Truancy
H   Normal concerns of childhood and adolescence

For each of the following cases choose the most likely diagnosis.

(26)   A 7-year-old boy will not go to school without extreme encouragement by his parents. When he is there he complains frequently of tummy aches and diarrhoea. He is a poor sleeper and usually tries to join Mum and Dad, as he is scared of the monsters in his bedroom. He dislikes going to birthday parties and will not stay over with his cousins unless Mum is invited, too.

(27)   A 10-year-old boy (the youngest of three children) had always done well at school until the family moved and he had to change to a new school. Now he is waking very early on school mornings with tummy ache and diarrhoea that resolve as soon as the decision is made for him to stay at home. He is

quite happy to go and spend the weekend with his best friend where the family used to live.

(28) A 33-year-old woman comes to see you to discuss her 14-year-old son. He has not been attending school at all over the past few months. He prefers to stay at home with his Play Station or hang around with friends in the park. He has never been academically very bright, but has always been quite well behaved and happy to look after the other four children when his mother goes to work.

(29) A 15-year-old girl has been causing concern at home. She has taken to locking herself in her room, listening to depressing music and reading poetry. When she does communicate with her parents it is usually in monosyllabic grunts. She is continuing to do well at school, and has a couple of close friends with whom she communicates constantly on her mobile phone and who seem to share her taste in music and verse.

(30) A mother brings in her 4-year-old son, who has been running riot at home for the past few months since his baby sister was born. She reports that he never sits still and that he constantly demands attention and entertainment. He attends a local nursery that has not reported any difficulties, but she thinks that he is hyperactive.

Theme: Murmurs

Options:

A   Ventricular septal defect
B   Aortic stenosis
C   Aortic sclerosis
D   Tricuspid regurgitation
E   Mitral regurgitation
F   Mitral stenosis
G   Mitral valve prolapse
H   Benign flow murmur

I   Aortic regurgitation
J   Pulmonary regurgitation
K   Pulmonary stenosis
L   Tricuspid stenosis

Which of the above heart valve/endocardial cushion defects fits each of the following clinical scenarios?

(31) A 4-year-old child has a 2-day history of runny nose and fever. On examination his chest is clear but he has an ejection systolic murmur.

(32) A 1-year-old with trisomy 21 presents to you with breathlessness when feeding and crying. On examination you hear a pansystolic murmur.

(33) A 76-year-old man comes for a routine insurance medical. He is fit and well and plays golf every weekend, but you hear an ejection systolic murmur that is loudest at the right sternal edge but does not radiate to the carotid arteries.

(34) A 45-year-old man presents with breathlessness. On examination you notice track marks on his arms, and he has a pulsatile enlarged liver and a pansystolic murmur at the left sternal edge.

Theme: Pharmacotherapeutics

(35) Calculate the correct dosage of cefaclor for a child weighing 12.5 kg. The dosing regime is 20 mg/kg three times a day and the suspension comes as 125 mg/5 ml.

How many millilitres should Mum give the child?

A   2 ml tds
B   5 ml tds
C   10 ml tds
D   15 ml tds
E   20 ml tds

Theme: Tympanic membrane

Options:

A Anterior
B Incus
C Light reflex
D Loft
E Malleus
F Pars tensa
G Pars flaccida
H Perforation
I Posterior
J Stapes
K Umbo

Label the following diagram from the above options.

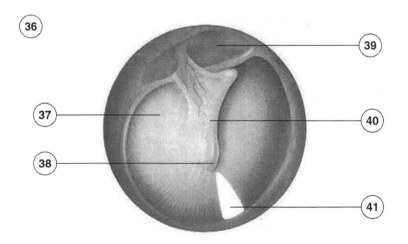

Theme: Menorrhagia

(42) How much blood loss is required to objectively diagnose menorrhagia?

A   20 ml
B   40 ml
C   80 ml
D   100 ml

Theme: Paediatric urological abnormalities

Options:

A   Immediately
B   6 months
C   1 year
D   18 months
E   2 years
F   3 years
G   > 5 years

At what age should each of the following be referred for corrective surgery?

(43) Hydrocoele.

(44) Undescended testes.

(45) Non-retractile foreskin.

(46) Inguinal hernia.

(47) Clinically likely testicular torsion.

Theme: Secondary prevention of stroke

(48) In the secondary prevention of stroke, the risks outweigh the benefits in which two of the following?

A   ACE inhibitors
B   Aspirin high dose
C   Aspirin low dose
D   Blood pressure reduction
E   Carotid endarterectomy for > 70% carotid artery stenosis
F   Cholesterol reduction
G   Warfarin without atrial fibrillation

Theme: Sildenafil contraindications

(49) Which two of the following are true of sildenafil?

A   It is contraindicated if the patient is on nitrates
B   It is contraindicated if the patient has a history of ischaemic heart disease
C   It is licensed for use in women
D   It is prescribable on an FP10 if the patient has had a prostatectomy
E   It is contraindicated in conditions that cause anatomical deformation of the penis

Theme: Dose of adrenaline for treatment of anaphylaxis

(50) What is the correct dose of adrenaline for treatment of ana-
       phylaxis? Choose one of the following.

A   10 ml of 1:1000 IM
B   1 ml of 1:1000 IV
C   1 ml of 1:1000 IM
D   10 ml of 1:1000 IV

Paper 4 Answers

Theme: Haematology

1. E
2. A
3. G
4. D

Discussion

There will be several data interpretation questions, but don't be thrown by them. They will provide reference ranges as would happen in general practice. Remember that they don't include red herrings, so clues such as ethnicity will point to the likely answers.

Theme: Employment law

5. C
6. B
7. A
8. F

Discussion

You will need to know a little about employment law. Look it up in Palmer's MRCGP® revision book and the *Oxford Handbook of General Practice*.

Theme: Mouth problems

⑨ B

⑩ H

⑪ J

⑫ D

⑬ E

Discussion

Often the questions are worded using quite formal medical phraseology. There will also be the odd merit point thrown in (epithelioma here).

Theme: Bone problems

⑭ F

⑮ D

⑯ C

⑰ B

Discussion

It is worth clarifying what happens to calcium/alkaline phosphatase, etc. in the common diseases you may be asked about (e.g. Paget's disease/osteomalacia). However, this can be quite confusing, and you would get the correct answer from the overall scenario in most of the questions, so don't fret over this.

Theme: Hip problems

(18) E

(19) F

(20) I

(21) A

Discussion

Hip infections may be seen in patients with prostheses or rheumatoid arthritis, or in the immunocompromised. They need to be referred for further investigation (bone scans are best), and require surgical drainage, antibiotics and bed rest.

Think about malignancies, particularly for the older age group and those with co-existing pathology.

Trochanteric bursitis is fairly common and can be managed with NSAIDs/physiotherapy, although steroid injections can sometimes help. Other lateral thigh pains are caused by fascia lata syndrome (inflammation of the fascia lata due to overuse or weak hip muscles) or meralgia paraesthetica, which is caused by compression of the lateral cutaneous nerve of the thigh as it passes through the inguinal ligament or where it goes through the fascia lata.

Avascular necrosis has multiple aetiologies, including sickle-cell disease.

Theme: Interpretation of trial data

(22) C

(23) M

(24) B

(25) P

Discussion

You will almost certainly get a question that involves a calculation like this. You are not allowed to use calculators.

Taken flu prophylaxis	Developed influenza		Total
	Yes	No	
Yes	1	274	275
No	12	263	275

Risk of developing influenza = number developing influenza/total in group.

Relative risk reduction (RRR) = risk of developing influenza without prophylaxis/risk of developing influenza with prophylaxis.

Absolute risk reduction (ARR) = risk of developing influenza without prophylaxis – risk of developing influenza with prophylaxis.

Number needed to treat = 1/ARR.

This part may seem hard to calculate, but going back to schooldays, 1/(11/275) is equivalent to 275/11, which you should be able to calculate without a calculator!

Theme: Psychiatric disorders of childhood

26̸ B
27̸ F
28̸ G
29̸ H
30̸ H

Discussion

Some knowledge of childhood psychiatric conditions is necessary, but it is just as important to determine where the 'psychiatric' boundaries lie before labelling naughty or adaptive behaviour as illness. There are strict criteria for diagnosing ADHD, namely that the three core features (inattention, overactivity and impulsiveness) have persisted for more than 6 months, are inconsistent with the developmental level of the child and are maladaptive. There must be impairment of academic or social functioning that is present in at least two situations, and some of these signs should have been present before the age of 7 years. The diagnosis has consequences in terms of labelling the child, medication administered and the way in which the child is subsequently managed both at home and at school.

Theme: Murmurs

31̸ H
32̸ A
33̸ C
34̸ D

Discussion

Some questions really are quite medical in nature, but you should be familiar with the presentation of heart valve defects as the primary point of contact for the patient. Do not get bogged down with complicated cardiac presentations – there are only a few murmurs that could come up. These would most probably be a stenotic valve, an incompetent valve or an endocardial cushion defect for a paediatric case.

Theme: Pharmacotherapeutics

(35) C

Discussion

Dose required in mg = weight of child × 20 mg/kg
                          = 250 mg.
Suspension is available as 125 mg/5 ml.
Therefore to obtain 250 mg you need 2×5 ml = 10 ml.

It is possible that simple calculations like this may come up in the exam, and note that the use of calculators is not allowed, so the numbers are likely to be very simple to work out. If you are getting into fractions and decimal points you are probably on the wrong track.

Theme: Tympanic membrane

(36) I
(37) F
(38) K
(39) G
(40) E
(41) C

Discussion

You may well be asked to label a picture of the eardrum, and also to identify photos of ear pathology (e.g. perforations, cholesteatoma, otitis media, etc.), so ensure that you are aware of what these look like.

Theme: Menorrhagia

(42) C

Discussion

This is the objective definition. Subjectively it can be defined as regular excessive blood loss in consecutive menstrual cycles in a woman of reproductive age.

Theme: Paediatric urological abnormalities

(43) D
(44) C
(45) G
(46) A
(47) A

Discussion

Paediatric urological abnormalities are an important part of child health surveillance, as many of them resolve in the first few years.

A foreskin should not be retracted before the age of 5 years. Circumcision is rarely required for medical reasons prior to this.

Inguinal hernias necessitate immediate referral due to the risk of bowel incarceration and damage to the testes.

Hydrocoeles usually resolve spontaneously by 18 months of age, and surgery is only required if they persist after this.

Theme: Secondary prevention of stroke

(48)   B and G

Discussion

The evidence that people with previous stroke or TIA should have their blood pressure lowered and be on low-dose aspirin is fairly well established. Further benefits are outweighed by the risk of haemorrhage if high-dose aspirin is given.

More recently, evidence is emerging that regardless of blood pressure or cholesterol levels, secondary prevention should include an ACE inhibitor and a statin (PROGRESS,[1] HOPE[2] and Heart Protection Study[3]).

The evidence shows that using warfarin for secondary prevention of stroke in people in sinus rhythm only increases the risk of haemorrhage, and confers no benefit over antiplatelet agents.

1   PROGRESS Collaborative Group (2001) Randomised trial of a perindopril-based blood-pressure-lowering regimen among 6105 individuals with previous stroke or transient ischaemic attack. *Lancet* **358**: 1033–41.
2   Heart Outcomes Prevention Evaluation (HOPE) Investigators (2000) Effects of ramipril on cardiovascular and microvascular outcomes in people with diabetes mellitus: results of the HOPE study and MICRO-HOPE substudy. *Lancet* **355**: 253–9.
3   Heart Protection Study Collaborative Group (2002) MRC/BHF Heart Protection Study of cholesterol lowering with simvastatin in 20 536 high-risk individuals: a randomised placebo-controlled trial. *Lancet* **360**: 7–22.

Theme: Sildenafil contraindications

 A and D

Discussion

Sildenafil and all of the phosphodiesterase inhibitors should be used with *caution* in cardiovascular disease, anatomical deformity of the penis, and conditions that predispose to prolonged erection.

They are contraindicated in patients on nitrates and those with hypotension, recent stroke, unstable angina and myocardial infarction.

They are prescribable on an FP10 in certain circumstances, including diabetes, Parkinson's disease, multiple sclerosis and prostatectomy.

Sildenafil is not currently licensed for use in women.

Theme: Dose of adrenaline for treatment of anaphylaxis

(50) C

Discussion

The nMRCGP® exam expects candidates to know how to treat emergencies. The other drugs used for anaphylaxis are oxygen, chlorpheniramine 10 mg IV and hydrocortisone 100–200 mg IV.

Note the difference between the cardiac-arrest dose of adrenaline (given intravenously) and the anaphylaxis dose (given intramuscularly), not to be confused with each other.

Paper 5 Questions

Theme: Benefits

Options:

A   Incapacity benefit
B   Severe disablement allowance
C   Invalid care allowance
D   Disability living allowance
E   Attendance allowance
F   Statutory sick pay
G   Child benefit

Which of the above benefits relates to each of the following?

(1) A 25-year-old with cerebral palsy causing a greater than 80% disability who has never been able to work.

(2) A 73-year-old man with severe dementia who needs help with all activities of daily living.

(3) A self-employed carpenter who needs 1 month off work following a work-related injury.

(4) A 42-year-old who has been unable to walk since a road traffic accident 3 years ago.

Theme: Urinary incontinence

(5) Which one of the following drugs has *not* been shown to exacerbate symptoms of urinary incontinence?

A Atenolol
B Bendroflumethiazide
C Cetirizine
D Diazepam
E Doxazosin

Theme: Concepts used in evidence-based medicine

Options:

A Prevalence
B Absolute risk reduction
C Attributable risk
D Correlation coefficient
E Hazard ratio
F Negative predictive value
G Null hypothesis
H Number needed to treat
I Odds ratio
J Positive predictive value
K Incidence
L *P*-value
M Relative risk
N Sensitivity
O Specificity

Which of the above best fits each of the descriptions below?

(6) The proportion of true negatives identified by a screening test.

(7) The likelihood of a person with a positive screening test actually having the disease in question.

⑧ The disease incidence in the exposed population minus the disease incidence in the unexposed population.

⑨ The disease incidence in the exposed population divided by the disease incidence in the unexposed population.

⑩ The statement that there is no difference between the two groups being studied.

⑪ The inverse of attributable risk.

⑫ The number of new cases of a disease in 1 year.

⑬ The probability of an outcome arising by chance.

Theme: Limping children

Options:

A Growing pains
B Hypermobility syndrome
C Osgood–Schlatter's disease
D Perthes' disease
E Septic arthritis
F Slipped upper femoral epiphysis
G Transient synovitis of the hip

What is the likely diagnosis for each of the following patients?

⑭ A 5-year-old boy has complained of pain in the hip for the past few days. He is limping consistently and there is a limited range of movement on examination.

⑮ A 14-year-old boy complains of pain in his knee, particularly after competing in athletic competitions. This pain resolves after a couple of days' rest.

⑯ A 13-year-old boy with a BMI of 29 has pain in his thigh and knee and a slight limp. Abduction and medial rotation of the hip are slightly limited.

(17) An 8-year-old girl has had pain in the hip radiating to the knee for the past week. It seems to be beginning to settle. She is systemically well, has no fever and is able to walk with a slight limp.

(18) A 7-year-old girl keeps waking in the night with aching knees. The pain is eased by massage, and she settles back to sleep after half an hour or so. She is otherwise well.

Theme: ECGs

Options:

A   Normal ECG
B   Sinus tachycardia
C   Sinus bradycardia
D   Atrial flutter
E   Atrial fibrillation
F   Ventricular fibrillation
G   Left ventricular hypertrophy
H   Right ventricular hypertrophy
I   Acute coronary syndrome
J   Old myocardial infarct
K   Left bundle branch block
L   Right bundle branch block
M   Trifascicular block
N   First-degree heart block
O   Second-degree heart block
P   Wenckebach phenomenon
Q   Complete heart block
R   Wolff–Parkinson–White's syndrome

What do each of the following ECGs demonstrate?

(19) A 64-year-old patient attends for an insurance medical. He is slightly overweight and has a family history of heart disease.

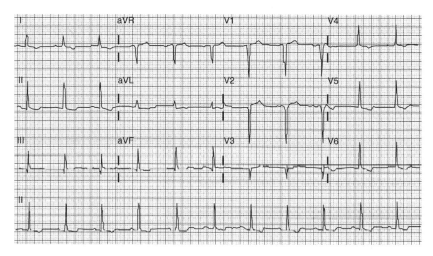

(20) An 80-year-old patient presents with a sensation of skipped heartbeats. She has a history of hypertension treated with diuretics.

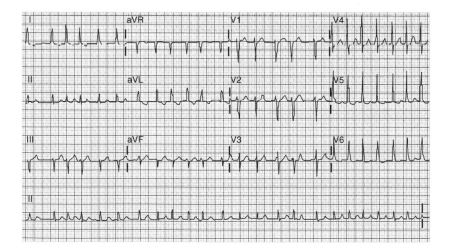

(21) A 40-year-old Afro-Caribbean man has recently been diagnosed with hypertension.

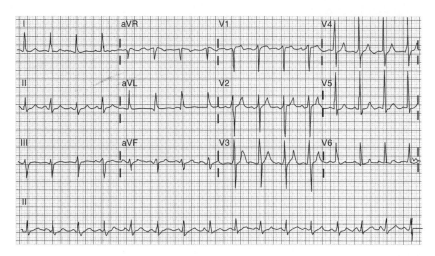

(22) A 71-year-old man presents with a 1-week history of significant fatigue and breathlessness on mild exertion.

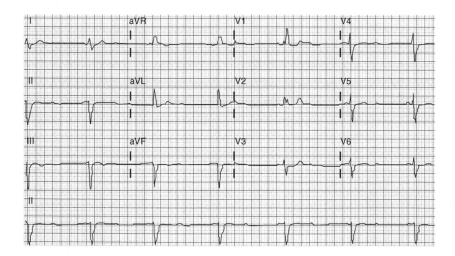

Theme: Vitamin/dietary deficiencies

Options:

A   Iron
B   Vitamin B_{12}
C   Vitamin C
D   Vitamin D
E   Vitamin K
F   Folate

What is the likely deficiency in each of the following examples?

(23)   A 30-year-old woman with vitiligo is found to have a macrocytic anaemia on a routine full blood count.

(24)   A 35-year-old epileptic patient who is well controlled on medication is noted to have a macrocytic anaemia.

(25)   A 27-year-old woman is feeling generally lethargic. Her haemoglobin is normal, but she does complain of heavy periods and her ferritin is low.

(26)   A 76-year-old with chronic renal failure complains of bone pain, and examination reveals a proximal myopathy.

(27)   A 4-year-old boy on the child protection register is brought to you for assessment. He has soft haemorrhagic gums and appears malnourished.

Theme: Practice leaflet

(28)   Which three of the following must be included in the practice leaflet?

A   Surgery opening hours
B   Surgery parking facilities

C   Disabled access
D   Baby-changing facilities
E   Date and place of doctors' first registration
F   Date and place of nurses' first registration
G   Length of consultations

Theme: Diabetes

Options:

A   Urine dipstick
B   Random glucose blood test
C   Fasting glucose blood test
D   Glucose tolerance test
E HbA_{1c}
F   Dietary advice
G   Commence metformin
H   Commence sulphonylurea
I   Commence glitazone
J   Commence insulin
K   Commence thiazide diuretic
L   Commence ACE-I
M   Commence statin

What is the next step in management for each of the following patients?

(29)   A 38-year-old patient comes in for a 'check up'. He is generally fit and well, his BMI is 24, and his blood pressure is 124/80. He mentions that his mother was diagnosed with diabetes at the age of 70 years.

(30)   A 60-year-old man was found to have a random glucose level of 7.2.

(31)   A 60-year-old diabetic is on 500 mg metformin three times a day. His annual HbA_{1c} comes back at 8.8, and you note that

last year's result was 8.5 (at which time his metformin was increased). He maintains that he rarely forgets his medication.

(32) A 58-year-old diet-controlled diabetic has persistent blood pressure readings of 155/94.

(33) A 56-year-old non-insulin-dependent diabetic is currently on glibenclamide. He has abnormal liver function (ALT stable at 100; normal range 5–35) secondary to chronic alcohol abuse, although he has been dry and hepatically stable for a number of years now. His HbA_{1c} has been creeping up and is now 9.2, despite maximum doses of glibenclamide.

Theme: Overdose

Options:

A   Arrhythmia
B   Convulsions
C   Heart failure
D   Kidney failure
E   Liver failure
F   Respiratory failure

What is the potentially fatal side-effect of each of the following drugs when taken in overdose?

(34) Ferrous sulphate

(35) Paracetamol

(36) Mefenamic acid

(37) Diamorphine

Theme: Asthma guidelines

Options:

A   Commence β_2-agonist as required
B   Commence low-dose inhaled steroids
C   Increase dose of inhaled steroids
D   Commence long-acting β_2-agonist
E   Commence interleukin-receptor antagonist
F   Commence oral steroids
G   Commence anticholinergic agent
H   Continue current management

For each of the following patient examples choose the most appropriate step in management.

(38)   A 5-year-old asthmatic girl is usually well on 100 μg beclomethasone bd and prn salbutamol. She presents with an upper respiratory tract infection, and her peak flow is 80% of normal.

(39)   A 25-year-old man has been using 200 μg beclomethasone bd and salbutamol as required for his asthma. Over the past few months he has been using the salbutamol daily and has been kept awake by a nocturnal dry cough.

(40)   A 15-year-old girl has been treated for exercise-induced asthma with a terbutaline inhaler as required. She is using this four times a week on average.

(41)   A 45-year-old man on 800 μg beclomethasone daily and bd eformoterol presents with a cough productive of mucopuru-lent sputum and shortness of breath on minimal exertion. His peak flow is 50% of the predicted value.

(42)   A 14-year-old boy has been getting a little wheezy when he does cross-country races. He tends to get protracted coughs postvirally in the winter, but is otherwise fit and well.

Theme: Drug side-effects

(43) Which one of the following drugs is known to cause sexual dysfunction?

A Ciprofloxacin
B Fluoxetine
C Ibuprofen
D Simvastatin
E Thyroxine

Theme: Antenatal testing

(44) Which one of the following cannot be identified by prenatal screening tests?

A Edward's syndrome
B Cystic fibrosis
C Hypothyroidism
D Beta-thalassaemia
E Fragile X syndrome
F Huntington's chorea

Theme: Visual field defects

Options:

A Left homonymous hemianopia
B Right homonymous hemianopia
C Bitemporal hemianopia
D Binasal hemianopia
E Tunnel vision

Which of the above visual field defects fits each of the following clinical scenarios?

(45) A 75-year-old man with non-rheumatic atrial fibrillation presents with a change in vision that occurred while he was driving, and resulted in his running the front passenger wing of his car into a lamp-post.

(46) A 30-year-old woman with post-pill amenorrhoea of 4 months' duration had this visual field defect picked up when she visited the optician this week.

(47) A 50-year-old man has noticed progressive loss of vision over the past few years. He initially noticed difficulty when driving at night. He recalls his father having similar problems in later life.

Theme: Cox II inhibitor guidelines

(48) According to the 2001 NICE guidelines, which two of the following patients should be prescribed COX II inhibitors as opposed to regular NSAIDs?

A   A 66-year-old with osteoarthritis but no other co-morbidity

B   A 58-year-old woman with polymyalgia rheumatica who is on long-term, low-dose prednisolone

C   A 42-year-old with a sports injury to their knee who has suffered from gastro-oesophageal reflux in the past

D   A 54-year-old woman with musculoskeletal back pain who has been using diclofenac prn, which is not working for her

---

Theme: Alcohol units

Options:

A   1
B   2
C   3
D   4
E   5
F   10
G   12
H   22
I   32
J   42

What is the unitary alcohol content of each of the following?

(49) A pint of beer.

(50) A bottle of vodka.

Paper 5 Answers

Theme: Benefits

① B
② E
③ A
④ D

Discussion

Benefits and who is entitled to them frequently come up as an MCQ question, and are worth learning. Note that the only difference between disability living allowance and attendance allowance is the age of the patient. Incapacity benefit is paid when someone is not entitled to statutory sick pay (i.e. they are self-employed). Invalid care allowance is the only benefit paid to the carer.

Theme: Urinary incontinence

⑤ E

Discussion

Diuretics, β-blockers, anxiolytics, sedatives and hypnotics have all been shown to worsen the symptoms of urinary incontinence.

Paradoxically, so have anticholinergics, antihistamines (due to antimuscarinic side-effects) and tricyclic antidepressants. The mechanism involved is exacerbation of urinary obstruction, thereby increasing the likelihood of overflow incontinence.

Theme: Concepts used in evidence-based medicine

(6) O

(7) J

(8) C

(9) M

(10) G

(11) H

(12) K

(13) L

Discussion

Ensure that you understand all of these concepts and that you can calculate them if required from basic data. Easy terms to confuse in exams are specificity and sensitivity, and incidence and prevalence. Make sure that you have an exam-proof way of remembering them.

Theme: Limping children

(14) D

(15) C

(16) F

(17) G

(18) A

Discussion

There is a pattern to limping children.

Condition	Age	Joint	Clinical features	Other features
Septic arthritis	< 5 years	Hip or knee	Holds joint immobile, systemically unwell	Emergency, requires IV antibiotics
Transient synovitis	2–10 years	Hip	Pain and slight limp, systemically well	Resolves in 7–10 days
Perthes' disease	4–7 years	Hip (10–15% bilateral)	Pain, decreased range of movement and limp	Urgent surgical referral for X-ray, bed rest with or without surgery
Slipped upper femoral epiphysis	10–15 years	Hip (20–25% bilateral)	Pain and limp often quite mild. Decreased range of movement	Can compromise blood supply, refer to orthopaedics
Congenital dislocation of hip	Congenital – may be noticed as toddler with limp if not picked up	Hip	Screened for in neonates/ developmental checks. If missed limp/waddle, asymmetrical leg lengths, falls	More common in females than males, increased in breech babies and those with a family history

Theme: ECGs

(19) J   Q-waves in V_2 and V_3 suggest previous antero-septal infarction.

(20) E

(21) G

(22) M   This ECG demonstrates Mobitz 2, left axis deviation and right bundle branch block. This often antedates complete heart block.

Theme: Vitamin/dietary deficiencies

(23) B

(24) F

(25) A

(26) D

(27) C

Discussion

There are a few common presentations of these deficiencies, and it is worth reminding yourself of them.

Theme: Practice leaflet

(28) A C and E

Discussion

There are certain facts that should be included in the practice leaflet, and all practices are obliged to provide them. Information that is expected includes the following:

● doctors – names, sex, qualifications, date and place of first registration

- primary healthcare team – details about the number of employed staff and the roles they fill, and whether the practice has students/trainees
- practical details – how to make appointments, clinic times, home visits, out-of-hours services, complaints procedure, geographical boundaries, access for disabled patients
- services – what is available (e.g. child health surveillance/minor surgery/family planning).

Theme: Diabetes

(29) A

(30) D

(31) H

(32) K

(33) J

Discussion

There are NICE guidelines (www.nice.org.uk) and recent NSF guidelines (www.doh.gov.uk/nsf/diabetes) on the management of diabetes but the clinical practice guideline on Type 2 DM (update) is currently being developed.

The healthy 38-year-old could be managed in different ways. Long-term lifestyle advice may well be sufficient for now, with the aim of screening him for diabetes in a few years' time. A simple urine test performed in the surgery may be enough to reassure him for now, and although it is not the most reliable screening test would probably be adequate. He could have a random glucose blood test, but this is more invasive and it is open to question whether it is necessary.

A random glucose value of > 6.9 warrants further investigation with a glucose tolerance test.

The next step for Question 31 is to add in a second oral hypoglycaemic medication, and the second-line drugs are the sulphonylureas. If these do not produce satisfactory results, they can be substituted with a glitazone. Beyond that, the next step would be insulin.

Recent trials (e.g. the UKPDS) have demonstrated that one of the most effective things you can do for your diabetics is to control their blood pressure tightly. The ALLHAT trial confirmed recommendations that thiazide diuretics are at least as effective as a first-line treatment for hypertension as more expensive treatments. There was no evidence from this trial to justify avoiding the use of thiazides in diabetics, and no evidence for the previously held belief that ACE-I protect against vascular disease independently of their effect on blood pressure. However, ACE-I are indicated if there is any degree of renal impairment.

The 2003 NICE guidance on glitazones suggests that they should be used in combination with another oral hypoglycaemic if other combinations are contraindicated or poorly tolerated. However, liver dysfunction is a contraindication to both metformin and the glitazones, so the patient in Question 33 would be better off trying insulin. Of note, recent evidence is emerging suggesting the benefit: risk ratio of glitazones remains unclear.

Theme: Overdose

㉞ E
㉟ E
㊱ B
㊲ F

Discussion

Although you would be expected to refer cases of poisoning to hospital, it is useful to know the potential problems. Iron tablets are often taken by inquisitive children, and in extreme quantities can cause hepatocellular necrosis. Tricyclic antidepressants are another common choice of overdose, and can cause respiratory depression, convulsions and arrhythmias. Long-term overuse of NSAIDs causes renal problems.

Theme: Asthma guidelines

(38) H

(39) D

(40) H

(41) F

(42) A

Discussion

The asthma guidelines are available at www.brit-thoracic.org.uk/ sign. This is a really good site with interactive case histories that are well worth looking at. They usually come up in one form or another, so it is worth having a thorough understanding of them.

Theme: Drug side-effects

(43) B

Discussion

This is a relatively common side-effect of the SSRI antidepressants in both men and women, and it can cause problems with concordance if not discussed with the patient.

Theme: Antenatal testing

(44) C

Discussion

Any genetic or chromosomal condition can now be diagnosed antenatally using samples obtained from amniocentesis or chorionic villus sampling. The Guthrie heel prick test is used to test for hypothyroidism and phenylketonuria 10 days after birth.

Theme: Visual field defects

(45) A
(46) C
(47) E

Discussion

This is a two-step question in that you need to work out the possible diagnosis before you can work out the clinical sign. The first patient is likely to have had a stroke, the second may have a pituitary adenoma, and the third may have retinitis pigmentosa.

Theme: COX II inhibitor guidelines

(48) A and B

Discussion

The main indications are as follows:

- over 65 years of age or significant comorbidity
- maximum doses of NSAIDs
- high risk of peptic ulcer disease (e.g. those with a previous history).

For full guidance, see www.nice.org.uk/pdf/coxiifullguidance.pdf

Theme: Alcohol units

(49) B

(50) I

Discussion

One pint of cider	4
One small sherry	1
One pint of beer	2
One glass of wine	1
One measure of spirit	1
One bottle of wine	7
One bottle of vodka	32

You should have a basic idea of the units contained in various alcoholic beverages.

Paper 6 Questions

Theme: Voice hoarseness

Options:

A Functional paralysis
B Hypothyroidism
C Laryngeal carcinoma
D Oesophageal reflux
E Overuse
F Sinusitis
G Viral laryngitis
H Vocal cord nodules

Choose the condition which best fits each of the following scenarios.

1. A 61-year-old smoker has noticed a gradual change in voice over the last 2 months.

2. A 58-year-old woman feels that her voice is much more croaky than it used to be, and has been generally tired for the last 6 months.

3. A 38-year-old opera singer is concerned that the timbre of her voice is changing.

4. A 32-year-old lecturer has a 1-week history of low-grade fever and malaise associated with hoarseness.

Theme: Developmental milestones

Options:

A   1 month
B   2 months
C   6 months
D   9 months
E   12 months
F   18 months
G   24 months
H   36 months

Choose the most likely age at which each of the following developmental milestones occurs.

(5)   Builds a tower of 3–4 bricks.

(6)   Speaks 3–5 words.

(7)   Sits with support.

(8)   Crawls.

(9)   Smiles.

(10)   Eats with fork and spoon.

(11)   Pedals tricycle.

Theme: Combined oral contraceptive

(12)   In which one of the following scenarios is the combined oral contraceptive pill absolutely contraindicated?

A   Father had an MI at the age of 44 years
B   A 33-year-old diabetic
C   Blood pressure of 145/93

D   History of migraine without focal symptoms
E   A 25-year-old who smokes 20 cigarettes a day
F   A 43-year-old non-smoker
G   A 38-year-old who smokes 20 cigarettes a day
H   A 29-year-old with a BMI of 32 kg/m^2

Theme: Certification

Options:

A   Mat B1
B   Med 3
C   Med 4
D   Med 5
E   Med 6
F   DS1500
G   RM 7
H   SC1

Choose the certificate that is most appropriate for each of the following patients.

(13)   A 44-year-old mechanic has a musculoskeletal injury to his back that would benefit from 2 weeks off work.

(14)   A 39-year-old woman with rheumatoid arthritis has been off work for 8 months. She has been sent form IB50 from the Department of Works and Pensions and has been told to get another form from her GP.

(15)   A 37-year-old woman who is 22 weeks pregnant wants to take maternity leave.

(16)   A 28-year-old woman discharged 3 weeks ago following a cholecystectomy rings asking for a sick note. The hospital have not issued her with one.

(17)   A 55-year-old man is suffering from alcohol-related problems and you have advised him to take time off work. He is

adamant that he does not want his employer to know his diagnosis.

(18) The district nurse asks you to fill in this form for a terminally ill patient so that he may claim attendance allowance.

Theme: Peripheral nerve lesions

Options:

A   Common peroneal nerve
B   Median nerve
C   Radial nerve
D   Sciatic nerve
E   Tibial nerve
F   Ulnar nerve

Which of the above nerves correlates best with each of the following examination findings?

(19) A claw hand deformity and weakness of abduction of the fingers. Sensory loss over the medial aspect of the hand.

(20) Weakness of flexors of the knee, and foot drop. Sensory loss on the lateral aspect of the lower leg.

(21) Inability to flex the toes, invert the foot or stand on tiptoe. Sensory loss over the sole of the foot.

Theme: Urinary symptoms

Options:

A   Anxiety
B   Diabetes mellitus
C   Hypercalcaemia

D   Infective cystitis
E   Post-radiotherapy fibrosis
F   Prostatitis
G   Pyelonephritis
H   Renal colic

Choose the most likely diagnosis for each of the following patients.

(22) A 64-year-old woman with breast cancer presents with intermittent abdominal pains. She also mentions that she has been passing large amounts of urine and drinking more than usual.

(23) A 26-year old man is seen as an emergency with a history of marked left loin pain for the last few hours. A urine dip is positive for blood.

(24) A 33-year-old woman asks for a home visit. She tells you that she has had dysuria for several days, and has now started to feel shivery and has right loin pain.

Theme: NSF guidelines

(25) Which of the following has not yet been incorporated into National Service Framework guidelines?

A   Mental health
B   The elderly
C   Coronary heart disease
D   Sexual health
E   Children

Theme: Shortness of breath

Options:

A   Occupational asthma
B   Fibrosing alveolitis
C   Extrinsic allergic alveolitis
D   Sarcoidosis
E   Cystic fibrosis
F   Pleural effusion
G   Pneumothorax
H   Bronchiectasis
I   Pneumonia
J   Chronic obstructive pulmonary disease
K   Asthma
L   Pulmonary embolus
M   Functional breathlessness
N   Panic attack

What is the likely diagnosis for each of the following patients?

(26) A 65-year-old man with a 40-pack-year smoking history presents with a history of breathlessness since flying back from Spain 24 hours previously. On examination he is pale and breathless, and percussion note is resonant but breath sounds are absent in the right upper zone.

(27) A 68-year-old lifelong non-smoking Asian man presents every few months with fever, cough, purulent sometimes blood-stained sputum and pleuritic chest pain. In between times he is quite well but has an occasional productive cough.

(28) A 36-year-old woman presents with increasing shortness of breath over the preceding 48 hours. She has some chest pain on inspiration. On examination she is slightly short of breath and her heart rate is 100. Oxygen saturations are 95% and her chest is clear. Her past medical history includes depression secondary to recurrent miscarriages.

29 A 35-year-old farm worker presents with malaise, cough and shortness of breath when crossing the fields. He finds that the symptoms increase during the course of the day. Bloods tests reveal a raised ESR and raised polymorphs.

30 A 60-year-old woman presents with wheeze on exertion. She has been monitoring her peak flow, which shows up to 10% variability, and her FEV_1 is 60% of that predicted. She stopped smoking 20 years ago, but had smoked 'quite heavily' in her youth.

Theme: Knee problems

Options:

A   Baker's cyst
B   Bipartite patella
C   Bursitis
D   Chondromalacia patellae
E   Dislocation of patella
F   Osgood–Schlatter's disease
G   Osteoarthritis
H   Recurrent subluxation of patella
I   Septic arthritis

What is the likely diagnosis for each of the following patients?

31 A 15-year-old girl has pain in the knee on walking up or down stairs. Pressing the patella against the knee causes pain.

32 A 72-year-old woman complains of pain behind the patella. She is a keen gardener and has been doing a lot of weeding recently. The knee is tender, and aspiration of the prepatellar fluid relieves some of the pain. The aspirated fluid is negative for crystals and bacteria.

(33) A 68-year-old man has a swelling behind his knee that is not painful, and he only notices slight discomfort when he bends down.

(34) An overweight 57-year-old woman has been experiencing progressively worse aching in both knees over the past couple of years. The pain gets worse towards the end of the day.

(35) A 12-year-old boy complains of pain below his left knee that is worse on playing football. He is tender over the tibial tuberosity, and straight leg raise against resistance is painful.

Theme: Abnormal liver function tests

Options:

A   Chronic alcoholic liver disease
B   Hepatocellular carcinoma
C   Cholestatic jaundice
D   Acute viral hepatitis
E   Autoimmune–haemolytic anaemia
F   Chronic active hepatitis
G   Gilbert's syndrome

What is the likely cause of each of the following blood test results?

	Normal range	Question number			
		(36)	(37)	(38)	(39)
Bilirubin (mmol/l)	3–17	84	100	87	24
Alanine transaminase (IU/l)	5–35	1250	195	47	80
Alkaline phosphatase (IU/l)	30–300	500	900	220	400
Albumin (g/l)	35–50	35	40	38	28
Haemoglobin (g/dl)	11.5–16	13.5	12.8	8	10.5
Reticulocytes (%)	0.8–2	1.6	1.4	10	0.8

Theme: Confidentiality

(40) In which one of the following scenarios would it be acceptable to break the patient's confidentiality?

A   An 83-year-old woman has declined treatment or investigation of a probable malignancy. She has not told her family, but her daughter calls you to ask what is going on, as her mother seems to be deteriorating rapidly

B   A 25-year-old florist continues to deliver flowers by car despite having had a grand mal seizure 6 months ago. You have warned her in writing that you will be obliged to notify the DVLA if she continues to drive, but she still refuses to stop

C   A 26-year-old woman had a termination of pregnancy but told her partner that it was a miscarriage. She had had IVF on the NHS because her partner had received chemotherapy and radiotherapy for a testicular malignancy when he was 16 years old. The partner is registered with you and books an appointment to ask what happened

Theme: Old age psychiatry or mental health of older adults

Options:

A   Anxiety
B   Dementia
C   Delirium
D   Depression
E   Paraphrenia
F   Normal adjustment reaction

What is the likely diagnosis for each of the following patients?

(41) A 75-year-old woman has been to the clinic several times over the past few weeks concerned that she is constipated. She had a normal colonoscopy earlier in the year, and in fact opens her bowels every other day. You have noticed her personal hygiene to be deteriorating and she has been losing weight. She admits to being kept awake at night worrying about her bowels.

(42) An 85-year-old man comes to see you with his wife. She reports that he has been becoming a little forgetful over the past few months, and yesterday used washing-up liquid to fry an egg. It is difficult to communicate well with him due to his poor hearing, but he does not engage well in the interview and scores 4/10 on the mini-mental test. Routine examination and blood tests are all normal.

(43) You are asked to visit an 84-year-old woman who has become increasingly confused over the past week. She has become incontinent of urine and is unable to recognise her daughter. She keeps asking for her husband, who died 20 years ago.

(44) A 75-year-old woman was widowed 2 months ago and has since complained of palpitations, breathlessness and tremor when she goes to the shops alone. She also has a feeling of apprehension, and difficulty in concentrating and sleeping.

Theme: Osteoporosis

Options:

A   Alendronate
B   Etidronate
C   Tamoxifen
D   Tibolone
E   Raloxifene
F   Parathyroid hormone
G   Hormone replacement therapy

H   Calcitonin
I   Calcium and vitamin D
J   Hip protectors

For each of the following scenarios select the most appropriate choice of treatments.

(45)   A 65-year-old woman had a DEXA bone scan demonstrating a T-score of −5 in both hips and spine. She had been on alendronate for 5 years when she had the scan. During that time she had sustained several fragility fractures.

(46)   A 48-year-old woman is concerned that she may develop osteoporosis, as her mother seems to be getting shorter as the years go on. She is still menstruating regularly.

(47)   A 42-year-old woman had a hysterectomy and bilateral oophorectomy 6 months ago after years of intolerable endometriosis. She is a slim lady who smoked for many years but stopped 6 months prior to the operation. Since the operation she has been having terrible night sweats.

(48)   An 85-year-old nursing home resident's daughter is concerned that her mother may sustain a hip fracture, as she has heard about the high morbidity and mortality associated with hip fractures in the elderly. The patient is slightly overweight, had her menopause at 53 years of age, and is a lifelong non-smoker.

(49)   A 63-year-old woman fractured her hip when she rolled out of bed on to a carpeted floor. She has had the hip fixed and is awaiting a bone scan.

Theme: Seatbelt exemption

(50) Which of the following is correct regarding the criteria for seatbelt exemption?

   A Women over 35 weeks pregnant

   B BMI > 35 kg/m^2

   C No criteria, it is at the doctor's discretion

   D For 1 month following abdominal surgery

   E Previous road traffic accident causing bruising to chest wall

---

Paper 6 Answers

Theme: Voice hoarseness

(1) C
(2) B
(3) H
(4) G

Discussion

Any persistent hoarseness lasting longer than 3 weeks should be referred in order to exclude malignancy.

Functional paralysis is an hysterical condition that is often seen in young women and is related to stress. It is a diagnosis of exclusion once other causes have been eliminated.

Theme: Developmental milestones

(5) F
(6) F
(7) C
(8) D
(9) A
(10) H
(11) G

Discussion

There is a high probability that this topic will be tested in the exam. Although there is an age range that counts as normal for each milestone, there are well-recognised averages. It will take a lot of time and effort to learn all of these, so it is worth memorising a few key milestones, and then an educated guess at the others can be made. A good basic mantra is 'one to walk, two to talk'.

Theme: Combined oral contraceptive

 G

Discussion

The recommendations for the combined oral contraceptive pill are to avoid it if two or more of the following are present:

- BMI > 39 kg/m^2
- blood pressure > 160/100 mmHg
- diabetes mellitus with complications
- smoking > 40 cigarettes/day
- abnormal lipid profile.

The combined oral contraceptive is contraindicated in patients with migraine with focal aura or a personal history of venous or arterial disease.

Theme: Certification

(13) B
(14) C
(15) A
(16) D

(17) E

(18) F

Discussion

This is another common MCQ question. An SC1 is the self-certification form needed to take the first 7 days of sick leave if the patient is not entitled to statutory sick pay. The DS1500 speeds up the claiming process so that terminally ill patients can receive their benefits more rapidly. Med 6 forms are used when a doctor feels that it may be harmful to a patient to have their diagnosis written on a Med 3 or 4. An RM7 is sent by the GP to the Job Centre to request a review of a patient sooner than the usual 28 or more weeks.

Theme: Peripheral nerve lesions

(19) F

(20) D

(21) E

Discussion

These are the common mononeuropathies that you will be expected to know. Remember also to remind yourself of the cranial nerves and associated conditions (e.g. Horner's syndrome, trigeminal neuralgia, etc.).

Theme: Urinary symptoms

(22) C

(23) H

(24) G

Discussion

Hypercalcaemia should not be forgotten as a cause of polydipsia and polyuria. Another condition to remember is diabetes insipidus.

Theme: NSF guidelines

(25) D

Discussion

The others have been issued as NSF guidelines. It is worth reading the main points of these and being aware of any new additions, but don't get bogged down by trying to learn each of the standards. A general overview will be more than sufficient.

The NSF for COPD is due to be published in 2008.

Theme: Shortness of breath

(26) G

(27) H

(28) L

(29) C

(30) J

Discussion

Remember that the examiners do not include red herrings – every bit of information has some significance. For example, the recurrent miscarriages are to make you think of antiphospholipid antibody syndrome predisposing to thromboembolic disease. It may be stereotyping, but if ethnicity is included it is usually a hint (e.g. Irish/Asian often used to suggest TB).

Theme: Knee problems

(31) D

(32) C

(33) A

(34) G

(35) F

Discussion

Knee pain is common in childhood and adolescence. This is often attributed to growing pains, but this can only be said of the aching pains that wake the child at night and are relieved by massage. There should be no residual pain the following morning, and examination is normal. Osgood–Schlatter's disease is usually seen in sporty teenagers who have pain and swelling over the tibial tubercle that resolves with rest.

Chondromalacia is due to problems with the cartilaginous surface on the posterior side of the patella. It is usually seen in teenage girls, and can be helped by physiotherapy to strengthen the vastus medialis muscle.

Theme: Abnormal liver function tests

(36) D

(37) C

(38) E

(39) A

Discussion

Some questions take longer than others, and if you are short of time you need to decide whether you can afford to answer a question like this and how confident you are about interpreting the blood test results. However, it is one of those subjects drummed in at medical school so that the information is stored subconsciously, to be 'taken out' at exam time. It can be simplified by thinking about acute vs. chronic and then pre-hepatic/hepatic/post-hepatic disorders.

Theme: Confidentiality

 B

Discussion

The GMC has provided a good guide to confidentiality issues (www.gmc-uk.org/standards) under the ethical guidance section. Essentially confidentiality is paramount for maintaining a trusting and successful relationship between doctor and patient. It may only be breached in the following exceptional circumstances:

- emergency situations in which breaking confidentiality will minimise the risk to life or health of the individual or another person
- statutory requirements, such as notifying the DVLA
- notifiable diseases
- court or tribunal summons
- adverse drug reactions.

Theme: Old age psychiatry or mental health of older adults

(41) D
(42) B
(43) C
(44) F

Discussion

Psychiatric diagnoses in the elderly are difficult and often fairly subjective. Question 43 could also be answered as anxiety, as this patient has all of the symptoms. However, these symptoms only become 'pathological' if they are prolonged or occur in the absence of a significant event or severely affect functioning. The diagnosis of dementia would be made after excluding organic causes. In the essay paper dementia is quite a favourite, as issues such as advanced directives, competence, confidentiality and autonomy can be raised.

Theme: Osteoporosis

(45) F
(46) I
(47) G
(48) I
(49) A

Discussion

The patient in Question 45 has severe osteoporosis that has not responded to a bisphosphonate. As a GP you would not initiate parathyroid hormone (PTH) therapy, but should be aware of the options available to a patient such as this who would benefit from referral to a specialist. PTH decreases vertebral and non-vertebral fractures by 50–65%.

Lifestyle advice and calcium supplements would be appropriate for the patient in Question 46. She is still young and so would not really fulfil the criteria for a bone scan at this stage.

HRT is a contentious issue. Obviously in women who have a premature menopause their lifetime exposure to hormones will not put them at risk unless they continue the HRT for many years beyond 'normal' menopause age. The patient in Question 47 is at risk of developing osteoporosis as time goes on, and since she is having menopausal symptoms she would benefit from oestrogen therapy. The recent trials (WHI/HERS) have not specifically looked at groups of patients like this, so we cannot say whether the HRT would put her at any increased risk of problems in the future.

The 85-year-old woman in Question 48 should ideally be on calcium and vitamin D (as should her co-residents). Hip protectors can reduce the risk of hip fracture in frail elderly women, but trials have been inconsistent and compliance can be a problem!

Sustaining a fracture from a minor injury should be regarded as osteoporosis until proven otherwise. Obviously more sinister causes need to be ruled out, but while awaiting the bone scan (which even if urgent can take several months) it is prudent to initiate a bisphosphonate. Alendronate and resedronate are the drugs of choice, as they reduce both vertebral and non-vertebral fractures by 40–50% (etidronate was one of the early bisphosphonates, and is not so good).

Raloxifene, a selective oestrogen-receptor modulator, decreases vertebral fractures by 36% and is also thought to decrease the incidence of oestrogen-receptor-positive breast tumours. There is a slightly increased risk of thromboembolic disease with this drug but it remains a good choice for patients with reduced T-scores and in the mid/early menopause, as they are more prone to vertebral than hip problems. It is recommended for the elderly, who are at greater risk of hip problems.

Tamoxifen increases bone mineral density, but there is little evidence of this translating to a reduced number of fractures, and there is an increased risk of uterine malignancies and thrombo-embolic disease. Data for tibolone are still awaited.

Theme: Seatbelt exemption

 C

Discussion

In view of the overwhelming evidence that it is safer to wear a seatbelt, there are no hard-and-fast guidelines as to who can be given an exemption certificate. It is therefore up to the doctor's discretion to decide who is eligible. An example of such a condition is a colostomy bag in a position where a seatbelt could obstruct it. Guidance and advice can be obtained from the DVLA.

Paper 7 Questions

Theme: Foot problems

Options:

A   Hallux rigidis
B   Hallux valgus
C   Hammer toes
D   Metatarsalgia
E   Morton's neuroma
F   Plantar calcaneal bursitis
G   Plantar fasciitis

What is the likely diagnosis for each of the following patients?

1. A 45-year-old woman complains of a sharp pain in the ball of her foot radiating into her toes when she goes out of the house. The pain is relieved when she removes her footwear and massages the foot. Examination reveals decreased sensation in the area that is causing the pain.

2. A 36-year-old traffic warden presents with a throbbing pain in his heels that has come on fairly suddenly after doing a lot of extra shifts at work.

3. An overweight 45-year-old man presents with pain in his heel, which is worse on rising in the mornings. On examination he is quite flat footed, and there is some pain on palpation of the inferior aspect of the heel.

4. A 67-year-old woman has a deformed first metatarsophalangeal joint that has resulted in the big toe deviating markedly

laterally, and she is finding that the joint rubs painfully on her shoes.

Theme: Fitness to drive

Options:

A   No restriction
B   24 hours
C   1 week
D   1 month
E   3 months
F   6 months
G   1 year
H   3 years
I   10 years

How long should you advise each of the following patients to refrain from driving?

5   A 56-year-old man with stable triple-vessel disease has just had his elective CABG and would like advice on when to start driving again.

6   An epileptic patient has recently commenced medication and wants to know how long he needs to be fit-free before he will be able to resume driving.

7   A 65-year-old woman had a TIA at the weekend. She has completely recovered.

8   An 18-year-old student passed out at a rock festival at the weekend. She was very hot, dehydrated and had prodromal symptoms prior to her blackout. She wonders how long she needs to wait before she can drive again.

(9) A 63-year-old woman is due to have coronary angioplasty and wants to know how long she must wait after the procedure before she can resume driving.

Theme: Adult psychiatry

Options:

A   Generalised anxiety disorder
B   Phobic disorder
C   Panic disorder
D   Post-traumatic stress disorder
E   Obsessive-compulsive disorder
F   Depression
G   Mania
H   Bipolar disorder
I   Schizophrenia
J   Personality disorder
K   Anorexia nervosa
L   Bulimia nervosa

Choose the most likely diagnosis for each of the following patients.

(10) A 30-year-old Somalian refugee has been having persistent nightmares and flashbacks to his time in Somalia before coming to the UK two years ago. He avoids members of the local Somalian community, and has sympathetic symptoms of sweating and palpitations, which he dulls with alcohol.

(11) A 21-year-old woman presents with restlessness and pressure of speech. Her ideas jump from one to another bizarrely. She has spent her entire student loan in the space of a week and has been very promiscuous, which is apparently totally out of character for her.

(12) A 25-year-old woman has an intense and persistent fear of being scrutinised and negatively evaluated by others. This fear

has been present since she was at secondary school, and results in avoidance of many social situations. It has become a problem recently as her role at work has been changed to incorporate attending and presenting at meetings.

(13) A 45-year-old man with fairly severe rheumatoid arthritis has been signed off work for 6 months as he is unable to cope with the pressures due to chronic pain. He feels extremely guilty about letting down his employers and being unable to provide for his family. He feels that his life is becoming worthless, and he has difficulty motivating himself to do anything. Even making simple decisions is becoming difficult, and his appetite is very poor.

(14) A 26-year-old man believes that he is too fat. He hears voices around him discussing him, and he thinks that the food he is given has been poisoned as part of a plot to reduce obesity in society.

Theme: Terms used in audit

Options:

A   Reliability
B   Criterion
C   Validity
D   Standard
E   Objective
F   Rationale
G   Effectiveness
H   Accountability

Choose the correct term to describe each of the following examples from an audit.

(15) Patients on repeat prescriptions of thyroxine under GP or shared care should have their thyroid function monitored at least yearly.

16. Ninety per cent of patients within the practice should have their thyroid function tested annually.

17. The results from the initial data collection were repeated by two different people and compared to ensure that they were consistent.

18. The initial data collection looked at all of the patients taking thyroxine and whether they had documented thyroid function tests taken within the past year in their records.

19. A review of the monitoring of thyroid function in patients on thyroxine has potential for improving clinical care, helping the practice to achieve higher standards in accordance with the new contract and, therefore, some financial reward if the gold standard of 90% is reached.

Theme: Respiratory tract infections

Options:

A Legionnaires' disease
B Tuberculosis
C Respiratory syncytial virus
D Rhinovirus
E *Haemophilus influenzae*
F *Streptococcus pneumoniae*
G *Staphylococcus aureus*
H *Pseudomonas aeruginosa*
I *Pneumocystis carinii*

What is the likely pathogen in each of the following examples?

20. A nursing home resident has developed a cough productive of mucopurulent sputum with a fever since a flu epidemic swept the home the week before.

(21) An intravenous drug user is very unwell with shortness of breath, cough, fever and pleuritic chest pain.

(22) A 1-year-old baby presents with coryzal symptoms that have progressed to an irritable cough and feeding difficulty. On examination he has an increased respiratory rate, and widespread crepitations over the lung fields with a wheeze.

(23) A 76-year-old with moderate COPD presents with a productive cough and on examination is found to have widespread wheeze.

Theme: Prescription charges

(24) Which two of the following diabetic products are available on FP10 prescriptions?

A   Urine testing kits
B   Blood testing sticks
C   Blood glucose monitors
D   Finger pricking devices
E   Glucose tablets

Theme: Urinalysis

(25) Which one of the following causes false-positive urine dipstick test results in the absence of red blood cells?

A   Beetroot
B   Myoglobin
C   Nitrofurantoin
D   Rifampicin

Theme: Visual loss

Options:

A   Vitreous haemorrhage
B   Cataracts
C   Chronic glaucoma
D   Diabetic retinopathy
E   Hypertensive retinopathy
F   Age-related macular degeneration
G   Migraine
H   Central retinal artery occlusion
I   Acute glaucoma
J   Retinal detachment

Choose the most likely diagnosis for each of the following patients.

(26)   A 75-year-old man with blood pressure of 168/100 complains of sudden loss of vision in his right eye. On examination, you note loss of the red reflex.

(27)   A 70-year-old man who smokes heavily complains of a 'curtain coming down across his vision' in the last 2 hours.

(28)   You are called to see an 83-year-old woman who has fallen at home. Her carers tell you that her vision seems to have been gradually deteriorating, and on examination you are unable to visualise the fundus.

(29)   A 69-year-old woman comes to see you complaining that although she can see 'around the edges', she is finding it increasingly difficult to recognise faces or read the newspaper.

(30)   A 45-year-old man comes for a routine fundal examination. You note microaneurysms, blot and dot haemorrhages and hard exudates. His visual acuity is normal.

Theme: Plasma autoantibodies and disease associations

Options:

A ANCA
B Anti-cardiolipin
C Anti-mitochondrial
D Anti-reticulin
E dsDNA
F Gastric parietal cell
G RhF
H Scl 70

Choose the antibody most likely to be related to each of the conditions below.

(31) Pernicious anaemia.

(32) Systemic lupus erythematosus.

(33) Coeliac disease.

(34) Recurrent miscarriage.

Theme: Neck lumps

Options:

A Branchial cyst
B Carotid body aneurysm
C Cervical rib
D Cystic hygroma
E Dermoid cyst
F Goitre
G Laryngocoele
H Lymphoma

I   Pharyngeal pouch
J   Reactive lymphadenitis
K   Sarcoidosis
L   Sebaceous cyst
M   Thyroglossal cyst

Choose the most likely diagnosis for each of the following from the list above.

(35) A 49-year-old man with a slowly enlarging single firm lump on the posterior border of the sternocleidomastoid, present for 3 months.

(36) A 79-year-old woman with a pulsatile mass in the anterior triangle.

(37) A 15-year-old with a midline lump which moves on protruding the tongue.

(38) A 19-year-old with a lump where the upper third meets the middle third of the sternocleidomastoid. It is non-tender.

(39) A 32-year-old with a diffuse smooth midline swelling that moves on swallowing.

Theme: Cervical smear interpretation

Options:

A   No action needed
B   Repeat smear as soon as possible
C   Refer for colposcopy
D   Repeat smear in 6 months
E   Take high vaginal, endocervical and chlamydia swabs
F   Treat if symptomatic

Which action is most appropriate for each of the following results?

(40) Borderline changes. Previously normal smears.

$\textcircled{41}$ Inflammatory changes.

$\textcircled{42}$ Mild dyskaryosis.

$\textcircled{43}$ Inadequate smear.

Theme: Squint

$\textcircled{44}$ Which of the following squints is the cover test demonstrating?

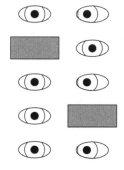

A Latent left convergent squint
B Latent right convergent squint
C Manifest left convergent squint
D Manifest right convergent squint
E Latent left divergent squint
F Latent right divergent squint
G Manifest left divergent squint
H Manifest right divergent squint

Theme: Secondary prevention in MI

(45) A 63-year-old man is discharged from hospital following a myocardial infarction. Which four of the following drugs have been accepted as essential secondary prevention to reduce mortality?

A Aspirin
B Atenolol
C Diltiazem
D Doxazosin
E Folic acid
F GTN
G Homocysteine
H Isosorbide mononitrate
I Losartan
J Ramipril
K Simvastatin
L Sotalol

Theme: Funny turns

Options:

A Vasovagal
B Postural hypotension
C Alcohol intoxication
D Cardiac arrhythmia
E Labyrinthitis
F Vertebrobasilar insufficiency
G Iatrogenic
H Hypoglycaemia
I Visual impairment
J Cerebrovascular accident
K Silent MI

L   Aortic stenosis
M Epilepsy
N Opiate toxicity

What is the most likely diagnosis for each of the following vignettes?

(46) A 23-year-old man is rushed to see you after collapsing after lunch at work. His colleague tells you that he became pale and sweaty on standing, slumped back into his chair, and his arms and legs twitched. He fully recovered within less than a minute.

(47) A 74-year-old woman has a history of falls. She tells you that it always starts with the room spinning and is worse on looking up at the ceiling.

(48) An 81-year-old man feels giddy on getting out of bed in the mornings. He is otherwise fit and well, although he has been treated for hypertension for many years.

(49) An 18-year-old collapses outside the surgery. You witness tonic-clonic movements and you note pinpoint pupils.

Theme: Infertility

(50) All of the following are indications for early investigation of primary infertility except for one. Which one is not an indication?

A   Female age > 30 years
B   Amenorrhoea
C   Previous pelvic surgery
D   Previous pelvic inflammatory disease
E   Abnormal pelvic examination
F   Testicular varicocoele present

Paper 7 Answers

Theme: Foot problems

1. E
2. F
3. G
4. B

Discussion

Most of these foot problems can be helped with well-fitting, cushioned shoes, foot padding and simple exercises (e.g. Achilles tendon stretching for plantar fasciitis). If they are persistently problematic, podiatry referral or even surgery may be indicated.

Do not be put off by the Latin names. If you don't recognise them you may well be able to work them out. For example, hallux (big toe) valgus (pointing laterally) clearly fits the bill for the patient with a bunion.

Theme: Fitness to drive

5. D
6. G
7. D
8. A
9. C

Discussion

The up-to-date DVLA regulations are available at www.dvla.gov.uk and www.gpnotebook.co.uk.

Theme: Adult psychiatry

⑩ D

⑪ G

⑫ B

⑬ F

⑭ I

Discussion

Remember the Schneidarian first-rank symptoms, of which more than one is suggestive of schizophrenia:

- thought withdrawal/insertion/broadcasting
- passivity phenomena
- thought echo (*écho de la pense*)
- voices referring to the patient in the third person
- primary delusions
- somatic hallucinations.

Theme: Terms used in audit

⑮ B This describes a measurable item of healthcare as a means of assessing the quality of that healthcare.

⑯ D The standard is the level of care to be achieved for a particular criterion.

⑰ A If a measure is used over and over again it should give you the same result. It is therefore reliable.

(18) C If the criteria are measuring what they are supposed to measure they are considered to be valid.

(19) F

A common cause of confusion is the difference between standard and criterion. It is also important to clarify in your mind what is meant by reliability and validity, as these come up in other aspects of critical appraisal.

Theme: Respiratory tract infections

(20) F

(21) G

(22) C

(23) E

Discussion

This is a bit medical, but you should be able to get at least 3 out of 4 with an educated guess. In general, infective exacerbations of COPD are *Haemophilus*, post-flu chest infections will be *Streptococcus*, intravenous drug users are prone to *Staphylococcus*, and pseudomonal infections are rare and tend only to be seen in chronic lung conditions such as bronchiectasis and cystic fibrosis.

Theme: Prescription charges

(24) A and B

Discussion

There seems to be no particular logic to this. Patients must buy their own blood glucose monitors, but are able to obtain the sticks for these on prescription. Lancets for finger pricking are available on prescription, but the mechanical devices that utilise these are not.

Theme: Urinalysis

(25) B

Discussion

Free haemoglobin is the other cause of a positive dipstick. The other items listed can cause a red discoloration of urine, mimicking frank haematuria, but the dipstick remains negative.

Theme: Visual loss

(26) A
(27) H
(28) B
(29) F
(30) D

Discussion

Remind yourself of the changes associated with hypertensive and diabetic retinopathy, as well as the classic presentations of the above conditions.

Theme: Plasma autoantibodies and disease associations

(31) F

(32) .E

(33) D

(34) B

Discussion

- These questions looks scary initially, but most of the answers can be worked out.
- Scl 70 is positive in systemic sclerosis.
- Anti-mitochondrial antibody is positive in primary biliary cirrhosis.
- RhF is positive in rheumatoid arthritis and polyarteritis nodosa.

Remember that these are not in themselves diagnostic, but can be highly suggestive of a particular condition.

Theme: Neck lumps

(35) H

(36) B

(37) M

(38) A

(39) F

Discussion

It is worth revising the characteristic features of these lesions, as they represent some of the surgical conditions of which GPs should be aware.

A cystic hygroma is a congenital abnormality. It arises from the jugular lymph sac and transilluminates brightly.

A laryngocoele is a pouch-like swelling in the neck found in wind instrument players. It is fairly rare, and can change in size as it fills with air.

Theme: Cervical smear interpretation

(40) D

(41) E

(42) D

(43) B

Discussion

Screening tests are always hot topics in primary prevention.

Risk factors for cancer of the cervix are as follows:

- age
- multiple sexual partners
- lower social class
- smoking
- no previous smear
- history of sexually transmitted infection, including human papilloma virus
- more than 5 years on the combined oral contraceptive.

Cervical screening is offered every 3–5 years to sexually active women between the ages of 25 and 64 years.

Further information can be found at www.cancerscreening. nhs.uk/cervical/index.html

Theme: Squint

(44) C

Discussion

Remind yourself of the descriptive naming of different squints. Variations on this question are relatively common exam questions.

Theme: Secondary prevention in MI

(45) A B J and K

Discussion

You will need to be fairly up to date for the long-answer paper. There are plenty of 'hot topic' books available. *Clinical Evidence* is a free publication which summarises recent studies, and the internet version (available at www.nelh.org.uk) provides references.

Theme: Funny turns

(46) A
(47) F
(48) B
(49) N

Discussion

Vasovagal attacks may mimic epilepsy, as tonic-clonic movements may occur, especially if the patient remains upright. Vertebro-basilar insufficiency is also known as brainstem ischaemia, and classically occurs on extension or rotation of the neck. In Question 48, it could be argued that this is iatrogenic, but the patient has been treated for hypertension for many years, and it is more likely that due to the ageing process his autonomic nervous system is unable to compensate adequately for postural changes.

Tonic-clonic movements are not diagnostic of epilepsy, but pinpoint pupils are highly suggestive of opiate toxicity.

Theme: Infertility

 A

Discussion

Female age > 35 years is generally accepted as an indication for early referral, not age > 30 years. The other indications are all correct. Note that in the investigation of primary infertility there is no indication to check thyroid function tests or prolactin levels if cycles are regular and ovulation is confirmed with a day-21 progesterone level.

Paper 8 Questions

Theme: COPD protocol

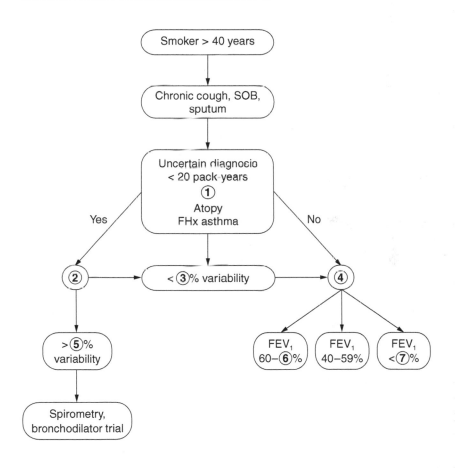

Please complete the sample protocol 1–7 from the following options:

A   Diurnal variation
B   Wheeze
C   Recurrent URTI
D   Eczema
E   10
F   20
G   30
H   40
I   70
J   79
K   80
L   Weight loss
M   PEFR qds for 1 month
N   PEFR bd for 2 weeks
O   Spirometry
P   Full lung function tests

Theme: Chronic kidney disease

Options:

A   1
B   2
C   3
D   5
E   10
F   20
G   25
H   30
I   35
J   50
K   70
L   75

M 80
N 85
O 90
P 95
Q 100
R 110
S 120
T 130
U 140
V 150
W 200

Please fit the correct numbers into the following statements concerning the management of chronic kidney disease.

General measures in the management of adults with chronic kidney disease include measuring blood pressure annually. Body mass index should be 20–⑧ kg/m^2. They should be advised to minimise dietary sodium to less than ⑨ mmol/day and restrict alcohol to ⑩ units/week for men and ⑪ units/week for women.

Medication should be initiated in patients with a blood pressure of ⑫/90 if there is no proteinuria, with a target of reducing the blood pressure to <⑬/80.

The threshold for patients with a urine protein:creatinine ratio >⑭ is 130/80, with a target of reducing the blood pressure to <125/⑮.

After commencing an ACE inhibitor or ARB, renal function should be checked within ⑯ weeks.

Recommendations are such that if the patient's serum creatinine concentration increases by ⑰% or GFR deteriorates by ⑱% secondary to commencing ACE-I/ARB, specialist advice should be sought.

The exception is with regard to the use of ACE-I in heart failure. According to the NICE guidelines it is acceptable to see an increase in creatinine concentration to ⑲ mmol/litre or a rise of ⑳% above baseline.

Theme: Contraception

Options:

A   Combined oral contraceptive
B   Condoms
C   Depot progesterone
D   Intrauterine system
E   Progesterone-only pill
F   Sterilisation

Choose the most appropriate type of contraception for each of the following scenarios.

(21)   A 17-year-old girl has had several prescriptions for post-coital contraception in the last few months. She tells you that she finds it difficult to remember to take tablets regularly.

(22)   A 21-year-old in a stable relationship requests contraception. She also asks if something can be done about her acne.

Theme: Teratogenic medications

(23)   Which two of the following medications are teratogenic?

A   Heparin
B   Fluoxetine
C   Penicillin
D   Roaccutane
E   Warfarin

Theme: Otalgia

Options:

A   Infective otitis media
B   Otitis externa
C   Temporomandibular joint dysfunction
D   Tonsillitis
E   Impacted wisdom tooth
F   Trigeminal neuralgia
G   Ramsay Hunt's syndrome
H   Chondrodermatitis nodularis helicis externa
I   Mastoiditis
J   Barotrauma
K   Furunculosis

Which of the above is the most likely diagnosis for each of the following scenarios?

(24) A 9-year-old boy returns from his summer holiday with a painful ear which is keeping him awake at night. He is unable to tolerate examination of the affected side.

(25) A 70-year-old man has had an excruciatingly painful lesion on the upper outer border of his left pinna for several weeks. He cannot lie on his left side at night.

(26) A 30-year-old man presents with a 2-day history of malaise, low-grade pyrexia and bilateral ear pain which is worse on swallowing. Examination of the ears is normal.

(27) A 7-year-old boy presents with a 10-day history of malaise, low-grade pyrexia and a painful discharging ear. Examination reveals tenderness behind the ear, but you are unable to visualise his tympanic membrane.

Theme: Childhood immunisation schedule

Options:

A	MMR	Pneumococcal		
B	Td	IPV	Men AC	
C	BCG			
D	DTaP	IPV	HiB	Pneumococcal
E	DTaP	IPV	HiB	Men C
F	DTaP	IPV	HiB	Men C
				Pneumococcal
G	HiB	Men C		
H	DTap	IPV	MMR	

For each of the ages below, choose the correct routine immunisations.

(28) 2 months.

(29) 13 months.

(30) 4 years.

(31) 4 months.

Theme: Mental Health Act 1983

Options:

A   Section 1
B   Section 2
C   Section 3
D   Section 4
E   Section 5
F   Section 7
G   Section 136
H   Section 137
I   Common law

Which section of the Mental Health Act would apply in each of the following circumstances?

(32) A 33-year-old schizophrenic man was discharged from hospital 2 months ago. He is becoming increasingly thought disordered. When you go to visit him he refuses to take any medication, and he has not eaten for several days as he has experienced voices telling him he must not eat.

(33) You visit a 45-year-old woman at the request of her husband. She was discharged from casualty the night before having taken an overdose of temazepam. When you see her she has a flat affect, expresses regret that the overdose did not work, and admits to plans for a second attempt when her husband goes to work the following day.

(34) An elderly patient has been admitted to your local GP unit with dehydration secondary to self-neglect since he lost his wife 4 months previously. He is trying to self-discharge, but during the week that he has been an inpatient he has been noticeably low. He does not interact with others on the ward, he has a very poor appetite, he wakes up in the early hours of the morning and he has expressed dismay at being admitted, as he would rather be dead at home.

Theme: Knee examination

(35) What is the most likely diagnosis for the following patient? A 26-year-old footballer twisted his leg with the knee flexed a few days previously. On examination, extension of the knee is limited and McMurray's test is positive. Choose the single best answer from the following options.

A   Collateral ligament injury
B   Cruciate ligament injury
C   Meniscal lesion

Theme: Headache

Options:

A   Subdural haemorrhage
B   Tension headache
C   Migraine
D   Glaucoma
E   Paget's disease of the skull
F   Cluster headache
G   Analgesic rebound
H   Meningitis
I   Temporal arteritis
J   Carbon monoxide poisoning
K   Subarachnoid haemorrhage
L   Space-occupying lesion
M   Cervical spondylosis
N   Extradural haemorrhage
O   Trigeminal neuralgia

Choose the most likely diagnosis for each of the following clinical histories.

(36) A 45-year-old smoker complains of recurrent headaches focused around his left eye, which becomes red and watery. They last for about an hour almost every day for a month and then disappear for several months.

(37) A 64-year-old woman has a 3-day history of a unilateral throbbing headache and facial pain. She tells you that it hurts to brush her hair and her jaw aches on prolonged chewing.

(38) A 36-year-old secretary is complaining of recurrent headaches for the last few weeks. She describes feeling as if a band has been tightened around her forehead. The headaches are worse in the late afternoon.

(39) A 43-year-old carpenter has a 1-month history of worsening headache. It is waking him up at night and is painful on bending over. He has also noticed a difference at work, as he cannot grip the hammer firmly enough.

(40) An 86-year-old woman has been suffering from headaches following a fall 2 weeks ago. Her daughter rings you as the patient is becoming intermittently drowsy and more unsteady on her feet.

Theme: Palliative care

Options:

A Macrogol laxative
B Dexamethasone
C Levomepromazine
D Diclofenac
E Oramorph
F Subcutaneous diamorphine
G Paracetamol
H Ondansetron

For each of the following patients choose the most appropriate drug treatment.

(41) A 62-year-old man with lung cancer has a 1-week history of pain in his ribs.

(42) An 88-year-old woman with colorectal cancer is started on MST for pain. Which other drug should be started at the same time?

(43) A 45-year-old teacher with a glioma presents with headache and vomiting.

(44) A 53-year-old man with liver metastases presents with nausea that is not controlled by metoclopramide.

Theme: Photosensitive rashes

(45) Which of the following can characteristically cause a photosensitive rash? Choose the three best answers.

A   Doxycycline
B   Ibuprofen
C   Paracetamol
D   Fluconazole
E   Erythromycin
F   Frusemide
G   Bendrofluazide
H   Metoprolol

Theme: Recurrent UTI

(46) Which one of the following interventions has been proven to be beneficial in the prevention of recurrent cystitis?

A Acupuncture
B Cranberry juice
C Double voiding
D Post-coital antibiotics

Theme: Ethics

Options:

A Autonomy
B Justice
C Beneficence
D Non-maleficence
E Consent
F Confidentiality

Which ethical principle is most relevant in each of the following scenarios?

(47) An 82-year-old man with severe dementia has an advance directive. His daughter would like him to have antibiotics for his chest infection.

(48) A 34-year-old man has had a recent seizure. You have informed him that he must stop driving, but he is continuing to do so.

(49) One of your patients is angry that his mother has to wait for her hip replacement. He tells you 'She can't even walk upstairs, but fit and healthy people are getting IVF for free'.

(50) A 14-year-old comes to you asking for contraception. She is very anxious that you will tell her mother about the consultation.

Paper 8 Answers

Theme: COPD protocol

1. A
2. N
3. F
4. O
5. F
6. J
7. H

Discussion

New NICE guidelines have been issued for COPD. Make sure that you are up to date with these.

Theme: Chronic kidney disease

8. G
9. Q
10. C
11. B
12. U
13. T

(14) Q
(15) L
(16) B
(17) H
(18) F
(19) W
(20) J

Discussion

An easy way to gain (or lose) marks is to fit the correct (or incorrect) word grammatically.

There is a website dedicated to revalidation which can be found at www.revalidationuk.info or www.gmc-uk.org/revalidation.

Theme: Contraception

(21) C
(22) A

Discussion

The intrauterine system has been shown to be equivalent in efficacy to sterilisation, is reversible, and negates the need for an operative procedure. It can therefore be recommended as an alternative to sterilisation and be used up to the menopause.

Theme: Teratogenic medications

(23) D and E

Discussion

Roaccutane is a vitamin A derivative and is severely teratogenic. Effective contraception should be used 1 month before, during and 1 month after treatment. Currently this is not compulsory, but soon European directives will dictate that women must be on the contraceptive pill prior to commencing therapy.

Warfarin can cause congenital malformations if it is used in the first trimester of pregnancy, and there is a danger of fetal and neonatal haemorrhage if it is used in the third trimester.

The other medications are not contraindicated in pregnancy, although heparin can cause fetal osteoporosis if used for prolonged periods.

The advice with regard to fluoxetine is to weigh up the need for the drug against the possible risks, although none have been reported in humans.

Penicillins are known to be safe in pregnancy.

Theme: Otalgia

(24) B

(25) H

(26) D

(27) I

Discussion

If examination of the external auditory meatus is painful, the diagnosis is likely to be otitis externa or furunculosis. Mastoiditis is rare, but one of the remits of the exam is to cover the serious conditions which mimic common problems. Question 24 may appear a little obscure, but it is possible to make an educated guess without wasting too much time.

Theme: Childhood immunisation schedule

(28) D

(29) A

(30) H

(31) F

Discussion

This should be a simple question, but its layout can cause confusion. It is worth reminding yourself of the immunisation schedules and the contraindications to vaccination.

Theme: Mental Health Act 1983

(32) C

(33) B

(34) I

Discussion

A question about sectioning seems to come up fairly consistently. There are many sources where you can find the criteria (e.g. www.gpnotebook.co.uk). Unless a GP facility has registered mental health status with the duty GP being the RMO, common law is the only way of detaining a patient who is considered unsafe until a Section 2 can be assessed.

Theme: Knee examination

 C

Discussion

You may need to know the names of some of these tests. McMurray's test involves flexing and extending the leg while applying pressure on the foot to rotate the tibia on the fibula. The idea of this is to trap the pieces of torn cartilage between the bones. The draw test is for cruciate ligament problems. The posterior ligament is damaged when the anterior tibia is hit (e.g. in car accidents). The anterior ligament is damaged when the tibia is hit from behind (e.g. in nasty football tackles). The anterior ligament is tested by pulling the tibia forwards with the knee at 90 degrees. The posterior ligament is tested by pushing the knee backwards with the knee at 90 degrees.

Ruptured ligaments require referral, as do meniscal tears, because they may require orthopaedic intervention. However, collateral ligament strains should resolve with rest, ice, compression and elevation initially, followed by physiotherapy.

Theme: Headache

(36)   F

(37)   I

(38)   B

(39)   L

(40)   A

Discussion

Headache is a favourite topic for EMQs, as the diagnosis is made mainly on the basis of the history. It is therefore a perfect subject for this type of question. Ensure that you are familiar with the distinguishing features of headaches, especially with the differences between subarachnoid, subdural and extradural haemorrhage, which are commonly confused.

Theme: Palliative care

(41)   D

(42)   A

(43)   B

(44)   C

Discussion

There are several drugs that are used specifically in palliative care and rarely elsewhere. Levomepromazine (Nozinan) is an example of this, and is a very effective anti-emetic which is slightly sedating. In Question 42 it may be argued that an anti-emetic should be given. These are not routinely started with opiates, as not everyone feels nauseated. However, nearly everyone becomes constipated, and it is good practice to start a laxative simultaneously.

Theme: Photosensitive rashes

(45) A B and F

Discussion

Many common drugs can cause this presentation. Again, do not spend ages pondering over this, as it is only worth one mark.

Theme: Recurrent UTI

(46) D

Discussion

According to *Clinical Evidence*, single-dose post-coital antibiotics and continuous prophylactic antibiotics are the only treatments proven to prevent recurrences. There is currently insufficient evidence to support the others, although results are suggestive of a benefit with cranberry juice and double voiding (going to the toilet again 5–10 minutes after passing urine).

Theme: Ethics

(47) A
(48) F
(49) B
(50) F

Discussion

It is important to know these principles, especially for the viva, but they do come up as EMQs. Several principles could be applied to these questions, but note that the question asks for the *most* relevant principle.

General index